SUPER Nutrition for WOMEN

Also by Ann Louise Gittleman:

BEYOND PRITIKIN

"Ann Louise Gittleman's *Supernutrition for Women* should be read by every woman (and the men interested in their health and welfare). This book is authoritative, easy-to-read, comprehensive, yet concise. It provides clear information about a health-promoting, tasty, varied and balanced diet. Such diets should restrict sugar and contain complex carbohydrates, essential fatty acids, vitamins, and minerals."

Dr. William G. Crook
Million Selling Author of *The Yeast Connection*

SUPER
Nutrition
for
WOMEN

*A Food-Wise Guide
for Health, Beauty,
Energy, and Immunity*

*Ann Louise Gittleman, M.S.,
with J. Lynne Dodson*

BANTAM BOOKS
NEW YORK · TORONTO · LONDON · SYDNEY · AUCKLAND

Note

The information contained in this book is intended to complement, not replace, the advice of your own physician, whom you should always consult about your individual needs. You should always consult with your own physician before starting any medical treatment, exercise regimen, or diet.

SUPERNUTRITION FOR WOMEN: A FOOD-WISE GUIDE FOR HEALTH, BEAUTY, ENERGY,
AND IMMUNITY
A Bantam Book / July 1991

Library of Congress Cataloging-in-Publication Data
Gittleman, Ann Louise.
Supernutrition for women : a food-wise guide for health, beauty, energy,
and immunity / by Ann Louise Gittleman, with J. Lynne Dodson.
p.   cm.
Includes bibliographical references and index.
ISBN 0-553-35328-4
1. Women—Nutrition.   2. Women—Health and hygiene.   I. Dodson,
J. Lynne.   II. Title.
RA564.85.G58   1991
613.2′082—dc20   90-22478
                                                                      CIP

Published simultaneously in the United States and Canada

Bantam Books are published by Bantam Books, a division of Bantam
Doubleday Dell Publishing Group, Inc. Its trademark, consisting of the
words "Bantam Books" and the portrayal of a rooster, is Registered in
U.S. Patent and Trademark Office and in other countries. Marca Regis-
trada. Bantam Books, 1540 Broadway, New York, New York 10036.

PRINTED IN THE UNITED STATES OF AMERICA
CWO   20 19 18 17 16 15 14 13 12 11 10

Dedication

*This book is lovingly dedicated to Edith and Arthur,
truly extraordinary human beings, who
also happen to be my parents.*

*And to Lena Falcidia,
my spiritual guiding light.*

Acknowledgments

My deepest thanks and appreciation go to my beloved mentors. To John Harris, my unforgettable high school English teacher for teaching me how to write; Hazel Parcells, N.D., Ph.D., for igniting my passion for healing; Nathan Pritikin for providing me a base from which to explore my own philosophy; and Paul Eck, D.C., for sharing his genius with me regarding the biochemistry of mineral balance.

Thanks also to my clients for being so supportive, loyal, and patient when I was away from the office on a research mission.

And thanks to my editor Leslie Meredith and literary agent Michael Cohn for his follow-through and enthusiasm.

I acknowledge the super women in my life who inspired me by their professional contributions and their own uniqueness: Ann Oliphant, Hanna Kroeger, Sharon de Buren, Sandy Berwick, Toni McMahon, and my right hand Lynne Dodson.

And to James, my super man.

Table of Contents

SUPER
Nutrition
for
WOMEN

ONE

Do Women Have a Fear of Fat?

Discovery consists in seeing what everybody else has seen and thinking what nobody else has thought.

—Albert Szent-Gyorgi

Susan is 38 years old and she is dieting—again. She couldn't count the number of diets she has been on since she first tried to lose her "baby fat" at age 13. A half grapefruit for breakfast, a salad with diet dressing for lunch, and broiled fish for dinner will help her reach her goal, she hopes. It seems to get harder and harder each time. It takes less time to regain the weight and more time to lose it, especially from around her waist. Desserts are her downfall—she rewards her daytime watchfulness with a "little treat" at night, Haagen-Dazs rum raisin ice cream. Susan is a chronic dieter.

Twenty-eight-year-old Pat works at maintaining nutrition despite a hectic life-style. She often reads articles on the latest food trends and is quick to incorporate them into her diet. Concerned about fat and cholesterol, she avoids oils, butter, red meats, and eggs. She eats shredded wheat with skim milk and bananas for breakfast, stir-fried brown rice with vegetables and soy sauce for lunch, and dines out frequently on pasta with meatless tomato sauce for dinner. Her one food vice is chocolate, which she craves, especially just before her period. Some of her friends call her a "nutrition buff."

At 18, Maryann is just beginning an independent life. One of the things she brought with her into her new apartment is her style of eating. Maryann is a "grabber"—a snacker who subsists on mini-meals as she rushes from one appointment to another. There are simply not enough hours in the day for her to sit down to three basic meals. Breakfast is a croissant and a cup of coffee, followed within a couple of hours by a diet cola and chips at her desk. Lunch with her coworkers is usually a hamburger, french fries, and a shake at a nearby fast-food chain. Dinner (if it's not pizza) has more variety thanks to the frozen food section. Fruit-flavored yogurts are her favorite snack.

These three women have different eating habits but share some common complaints. They feel tired much of the time; they are irritable and often feel cold; they seldom sleep soundly through the night; they have various aches and pains which seem to have no cause; they are the first to get the season's colds; and vaginal infections, menstrual cramps, and bloating plague them every month. A visit to the doctor rules out a medical problem, so they think it must be "stress," "that time of life," "getting old," or "hormonal readjustment"—in any case, just something to live with. The longer they maintain their diet styles, the greater the likelihood that they will develop anemia, heart disease, cancer, osteoporosis, premenstrual syndrome, and arthritis.

Susan, Pat, and Maryann are fictionalized women, but they represent the three basic female eating patterns I have observed while reviewing more than 7,000 diet histories throughout my career—as the chief dietitian of the Pediatric Clinic at Bellevue Hospital in New York City; nutritionist for the U.S. Department of Agriculture (U.S.D.A.) Women, Infants, and Children Food Program in New Haven, Connecticut; nutrition consultant for the first holisitic medical group in Connecticut, Deep Brook Associates; and later as nutrition director at the Pritikin Longevity Center in Santa Monica, California, and consultant to medical doctors, corporations, and environmental health clinics.

The chronic dieter, nutrition buff, and grabber are three basic female eating types I have noted over the past two decades all over the country. These eating types have also been the focus of attention for U.S.D.A. nutrition educators and other researchers throughout the country for two decades, and they seem to cross economic and age categories. They can be identified in the diet histories of patients I counseled as far back as the late 1970s in the inner city of New Haven, Connecticut, as well as of patients in Marin County, California, whom I counseled in the late 1980s.

Whether in private practice, at hospitals, or in public health clinics, I have always required that my clients keep a food diary, recording what, when, and where they eat and drink, as well as their emotions at the time. By reviewing this record of total food intake over a period of three to seven days, I have been able to gauge their current eating habits.

Through my counseling I have evaluated the health impact of these eating styles and the concerns that have motivated women to adopt them in the first place. I have identified the potential health hazards of such eating patterns, and I have found food solutions that are nutritious, delicious, and convenient, whether at home or on the go.

Chronic Dieter

Let's begin with a little background on the chronic dieter who is dieting (again) for weight loss. A recent National Health Interview Survey found almost half of American adult women were dieting at any one time.

In my own counseling experience, the majority of clients who have come to see me over the years have wanted to lose weight. Many had already tried the most popular diets, including Stillman, Atkins, Pritikin, and most recently, Fit for Life, or the new liquid protein fast known as very low calorie diets (VLCD). Were these women on the right track? The answer is yes and no. There are basically only two ways to lose weight: burn more calories with exercise, or take in fewer calories with diet. Most women choose this second way.

Furthermore, most of my clients tried to speed up the weight loss process by skipping meals, believing that by eating even less they would lose more weight faster.

As you read this, an estimated 65 million Americans are deliberately starving themselves in an effort to conform to society's and their own ideal body image. Twice as many women are likely to diet as men. Even women who are underweight are trying to eat less—some 3 million of them. In fact, some health authorities believe only 20 percent of women eat "normally," without dieting.

Yet the National Center for Health Statistics estimates that 27 percent of women over age 20 are substantially overweight. A study by the Centers for Disease Control has found that nearly 8 percent of women put on more than 30 pounds between ages 25 and 35. Fatness has been increasing steadily over the past three decades in the United States: since the 1960s, the number of obese women has increased by at least 4.2 million. We spend $20 billion annually on diet books, pills, foods, and gimmicks, but at the same time we are consuming candy in record amounts. One study of dieters found that they are eating 30 percent more muffins, 46 percent more chocolate bars, and twice as many croissants as they did in the early 1980s.

I've often speculated that fatness is on the increase *because* of our preoccupation with dieting. Eating, not skipping meals, elevates the body's metabolic rate. In fact, as my former chronic dieters can testify, simply eating three meals a day can burn up to 10 percent more calories. This translates into 200 more burned calories for most women on a daily basis.

Taking in fewer calories usually means taking in fewer nutrients as well. The U.S.D.A. 1986 study of food consumption found that women got significantly less than the recommended daily allowances (RDAs) of seven nutrients: vitamins B_6 and E, calcium, magnesium, iron, folic acid, and zinc.

Yo-Yo Dieting Risks

The effects of these schizophrenic eating habits have recently become the subject of serious research. At the University of Pennsylvania and elsewhere, scientists are studying what has become known as the Yo-Yo Syndrome. Their conclusion—dieting can make you fat!

The Yo-Yo Syndrome refers to cycles of weight gain

and loss from dieting. Unable to distinguish between famine and dieting, the body reacts to fewer calories with inherent defenses, biological mechanisms designed to withstand starvation and protect the species. Your basal metabolic rate actually slows down. Since this rate accounts for 60 to 75 percent of the energy used by the body—for routine functions like breathing and cell repair—its slowdown calls a halt to weight loss.

In addition, the body becomes more efficient in *storing* fat. Enzymes are complex proteins that regulate the body's chemical processes. One of them, called lipase, predigests dietary fat before it enters the intestine and thus makes the fat easier to digest and store. In yo-yo dieters, this enzyme becomes more active in preparing fat to be stored in fat cells.

These metabolic changes also cause a woman's body to gain weight faster and hold on to it once calorie intake returns to normal.

Kelly Brownell, Ph.D., and the researchers of the Weight Cycling Project have seen other hazards in yo-yo dieting in their preliminary data:

- Women who yo-yo diet may redistribute their body fat from the thighs and hips (the predominant location on the female body) to the abdomen. The fatter a person is from the waist up, the greater the risk for diabetes and heart disease.

- Yo-yo dieting may increase the body's fat-to-lean tissue ratio. Women may lose considerable muscle tissue while dieting, but tend to regain it as fat.

- Yo-yo dieters may find their desire for fatty foods, many of which are unhealthful, increases.

- Additional risk from heart disease may come from the cycling of weight up and down. The long-term Framingham Heart Study, which has monitored more than 5,000 people for almost 40 years, has found that people who raised their body weight 10 percent increased their risk of coronary artery disease by 30 percent. On the other hand, if they lost 10 percent of body weight, they decreased their risk by only 20 percent, for a net increase of 10 percent in risk every loss-gain cycle.

Now you can understand why every time you diet, it gets harder and harder to lose weight. It is not just common sense, but biochemical fact, that changing eating habits *gradually* (combined with exercise) is the only effective way to lose weight.

The Chronic Dieter and Energy-Sapping Diets

In addition to metabolic slowdown, diets that reduce calories also often exclude entire categories of foods. This sets women up for nutritional deficiencies. Red meat is a good case in point. A diet of fruits, vegetables, grains, and fish and poultry may be high in vitamins A and C and protein, but significantly deficient in blood-building iron, vitamin B_{12}, and the trace mineral zinc. These deficiencies can bring on anemia, asthma, hair loss, and psoriasis.

Women who feel deprived by low-calorie diets are more likely to cheat by devouring high-calorie, vitamin-deficient treats like gourmet cookies and rich desserts. How many times have I noted a coconut chocolate chip cookie, butternut ice cream, or raspberry tart on the food diary of a chronic dieter who has sworn off red meat, but treats herself to a fattening reward. These high-sugar, high-saturated-fat foods may lead to anemia, osteoporosis, menstrual problems, and dry skin and hair by displacing more substantial foods in the diet.

The Nutrition Buff

What about nutrition-conscious women like Pat? I have worked with hundreds of "Pats," who comprise the second largest group of patients consulting me for health problems. They think they are keeping fit and healthy by their watchfulness. Unfortunately, this is not the case for many of them.

Redbook, Glamour, and other women's magazines that regularly poll their readers find that women say they are eating more poultry and fish, reading labels for nutrition information, and snacking on fruit.

Yet industry sales figures and national food consumption studies give a different view. The U.S.D.A. found no increase in the percentage of women serving fish or fruits on a given survey day in 1977 and in 1986. As I pointed out earlier, the same study found women getting less than recommended amounts of vitamins B_6 and E, calcium, magnesium, iron, folic acid, and zinc, all critical to a woman's good health and optimum reproductive function.

Fat Deception

Many women are concerned about fats and, in particular, cholesterol. The late nutrition pioneer Nathan Pritikin, the American Heart Association, the Surgeon General, food editors all over the country, and even many food manufacturers urge a significant reduction of dietary fat as the way to health—to 30 percent of calories, down from the 40-plus percent most Americans consume. The Pritikin diet, with its emphasis on only 5–10 percent of calories from fats, has convinced millions that fats are bad and linked with various degenerative diseases, particularly heart disease, America's number one killer.

My "Pats" have been classic. They are so anti-fat that they have not only sworn off every nut, seed, and avocado on the planet, but they'd rather be caught dead than use a drop of oil on their foods. Some of these women have become *too* lean from their obsessive dieting.

One of my clients, 33-year-old Gina, was a strong advocate of the low-fat, high-complex-carbohydrate diet because she believed it was the ideal diet for athletes. She ran almost five miles a day. When she consulted me because her periods had stopped, I explained that in addition to her extremely low-fat diet (fat makes hormones, as you will read later), her excessive exercise may have further reduced her body's fat stores and disrupted hormonal function, which ultimately reduced the estrogen levels in her body. Overexercise causes the body to stop making estrogen and utilize calcium, which is estrogen dependent! I suggested that she decrease her running by one half, to two and one-half miles a day, and that she gain at least five pounds. I also told her to add one or two tablespoons of safflower or olive oil to her daily diet. As it turned out, her period returned when she had regained only three pounds.

What advocates of the low-fat, high-carbohydrate diet overlook is the evidence about the crucial—and positive—role some fats play in the diet. Women like Gina and others, who want to be thin but fertile, suffer the most from this nutritional one-sidedness.

As I will describe more fully in Chapter Three, certain vitamins must have fat present in order to be dissolved and absorbed into the body. Essential fatty acids (EFAs) play a positive role in a myriad of female reproductive disorders like premenstrual syndrome, viral and yeast infections, and infertility, as well as food allergy and immune disorders. EFAs strengthen cell membranes, which are our bodies' first defense against infections. Essential fats are also vital to healthy skin, hair, and nails (they are often added to hair and skin care products for topical application). Most important, essential fats are needed to form the hormonelike substances prostaglandins, which control the body's immune, cardiovascular, reproductive, and central nervous systems. Without prostaglandins (and the essential fats necessary for their production), our blood does not clot, tumors grow unchecked, cells become inflamed, and allergies rage out of control.

Fat and Calcium

The right kind of fat is necessary for calcium availability in the soft tissues and to promote calcium elevation in the bloodstream—so that muscles contract properly and maintain their tone, nerves function smoothly, blood clots when needed, and bones and teeth remain strong and healthy. Women who believe they are getting enough calcium through diet and supplements may be sabotaging themselves if they do not include enough of the right oils in their diets.

The Grabber Versus Grazer

Maryann, our mini-meal eater and constant snacker, is fast becoming the norm in women's eating habits. Visit almost any major American shopping mall—shops selling chocolate chip cookies, European chocolates, croissants, and gourmet ice cream have joined the dress, shoe, and department stores as mall staples.

For many teenagers like Maryann, junk-food snacks and fast-food meals form a habit that is carried into adulthood. Fast-food restaurants make up almost 50 percent of all eating places in the United States, with more than 140,000 in operation. In fact, McDonald's opens two new restaurants every day of the year.

Unlike sugar-laden junk food, which by definition has almost no food value, fast food does have some nutritional value. But it lacks several key vitamins and minerals—vitamins A, B_1, and C, and calcium, in particular—and a steady diet of fast food can be hazardous. The excesses of saturated fat, sodium, calories, and even sugar add to the problem.

The typical meal of hamburger-fries-shake (not a milk shake, since it contains almost no milk) weighs in at almost 1,000 calories. Individuals who select the fish sandwich thinking it's healthier are in for a surprise—processing, breading, and deep-fat frying turn the wholesome low-fat fish into a high-fat food:

Comparison of Two Fast-Food Staples

	Burger King Whopper	Burger King Whaler
Calories	630	486
Protein	26 grams	18 grams
Carbohydrates	50 grams	64 grams
Fats	36 grams	46 grams
Sodium	990 milligrams	735 milligrams

Source: Adapted from *Fat-Proofing Your Children,* by Vicki Lansky (New York: Bantam Books, 1988).

Women who eat on the run have created a booming market for convenience foods as well. Retail sales of frozen dinners and entrees were over $4.5 billion in 1986. Joining the three-course dinners are single-serving vegetable side dishes, gourmet entrees from around the world, and single-serving desserts.

Undeniably convenient and appealing, today's frozen foods achieve much of their appeal at the cost of healthfulness—the average frozen food entree is over 50 percent fat and some may contain over half of a woman's recommended daily sodium intake (1,100–3,300 milligrams), as this chart of just a few products highlights:

Frozen Dinners and Entrees
(average over product line)

Brand (serving size)	Fat (percent of cals)	Calories	Sodium (mg)
La Choy Dinners (12 oz)	10	243	1,822
Light & Elegant (9 oz)	19	259	880
Lean Cuisine (10 oz)	28	260	978
Weight Watchers (10 oz)	35	277	1,051
Armour Dinner Classics (11 oz)	39	391	1,339
Swanson 4-part Dinners (12 oz)	40	483	1,154
Le Menu (11 oz)	42	398	1,001
Budget Gourmet (10 oz)	43	373	849

Brand (serving size)	Fat (percent of cals)	Calories	Sodium (mg)
Stouffer's Entrees (9 oz)	46	343	1,130
Old El Paso (na)	55	359	623

Source: © 1989 CSPI. Reprinted from *Nutrition Action Healthletter* (1501 16th Street, N.W., Washington, D.C. 20036-1499. $19.95 for 10 issues.)

Maryann's problem as a grabber is related less to her pattern of eating than to what she eats. It is not necessary to eat three "square meals" a day to get the healthy balance of nutrients and calories you need. Mini-meal eaters, or grazers, who select wisely benefit not only in good health but also in weight control. In fact, a study reported in the *Journal of the American Medical Association* found that women who ate one large meal a day instead of several small ones were 25 times more likely to store fat. The constant nibbling of the women who ate several small meals stimulated their bodies' brown fat, a special fat-burning tissue that produces body heat by burning calories rather than storing the calories as fat cells. This meant that the women's bodies stored less fat, their metabolism rose as their food intake rose, and they lost weight.

I was first introduced to the concept of grazing (as opposed to grabbing!) while working as the director of nutrition at the Pritikin Longevity Center. In the early 1980s, the Center served six mini-meals a day. This concept of constant feeding was so integral to the program, but avant garde at the time, that the meals and food timings were printed on T-shirts, which all the participants wore.

These mini-meals included many healthy foods, but lacked one key element—fat. Like the others on the program, I was constantly grazing because I was always hungry. The fat-free meals never left me satisfied. I can remember downing bowl after bowl of oatmeal, wheat berries, or steamed barley before my morning lectures in order to feel full. In fact, the Pritikin fat-free regimen kept me from using even a bit of butter on my grains, so I was always hungry. (Fat slows down digestion; it takes at least two more hours for food to digest with fat than without it. Hunger is therefore retarded when a small amount of fat is added to the meals.) Thus, for Pritikin participants, grazing was a necessity, almost an obsession.

Grazing is no longer considered avant garde, but has become part of the current nutritional prescription of sound dietary practice. If grazers choose wisely and include fats, carbohydrates, and protein in balanced mini-meals, they can avoid the trap of becoming either a grabber or a Pritikin-style grazer.

The Sour Side of Sugar

All three eating styles share one potential pitfall—the lure of sugar in its many forms.

Desserts and sugar-laden snacks tempt a woman to choose happiness over health. Women who carefully monitor their food intake all day might indulge in a rich dessert reward at night—what one observer has termed the "Lean Cuisine/Dove Bar mentality." Restaurants report an ever-increasing demand for the richest desserts they can produce. Nearly 40 percent of Americans eat ice cream often. In fact, Americans average 15 quarts per person per year. Gourmet brands, which are growing in popularity, get their richness from a recipe that is more than double the fat content of less expensive brands (a half cup of Haagen-Dazs vanilla ice cream contains 260 calories and 17 grams of fat; Breyers has 150 calories and 8 grams of fat).

These cravings are a complex mix of physiological and psychological factors, not yet fully understood. We know that fat in the diet gives a sense of fullness, so that when the body is fat-starved, it sends insistent hunger messages. Good-tasting foods, including sweets, stimulate the palate and bring pleasure. There is a chemical basis for this in the mood-altering brain chemicals that are triggered by eating carbohydrates (cookies, cakes, muffins). In addition, many of us carry from childhood the "knowledge" that the reward for good behavior is a cookie, not a carrot.

Our sweet tooth contributes directly and indirectly to osteoporosis, premenstrual syndrome, excess weight, coronary artery disease, and cancer. Excess sugar is converted in the body to nonessential fatty acids (such as saturated fats) and cholesterol. One study by the U.S.D.A. found that individuals who consumed 30 percent of their calories from sugar (slightly more than the typical American diet) developed significantly higher levels of cholesterol and triglycerides (fats) in their blood than did control subjects who had wheat starch substituted for the sugar.

Sugar consumption adversely affects the calcium-phosphorus balance so crucial to effective calcium absorption. If calcium levels in the blood are inadequate, calcium is drawn from bones and teeth, contributing to the development of osteoporosis and dental disease. Furthermore, calcium is essential for proper muscle function; deficiencies lead to muscle cramps, including those associated with menstruation. A recent American study has found that calcium also helps neutralize bile acids and fatty acids which can irritate the bowel and contribute to the formation of colon cancer.

Eating sugar with fat, as in ice cream, doughnuts and other baked goods, and butter-rich chocolates, causes the body to store fat more readily, rather than burning it for energy (see Chapter Four).

Is There a Solution?

Many women are becoming more aware of how diet affects their bodies. They are making the connection between what they eat and how they feel. Many of my clients are eating some red meat, and more fish and vegetables. They're eating less salt and cutting back on their sugar habit. But this is only the beginning for the food-wise woman. We need to truly support female health. We need to know how chemical imbalances create a climate for disease and unhealthfulness. We must learn to protect the crucial "female minerals" from inhibitors—sugar, caffeine, soft drinks, and saturated fats—and to return valuable food staples to our diet, including lean red meat and eggs. We need to know the "good" side of cholesterol and dietary fats and learn to incorporate them into a balanced diet.

All of this can be done without exotic foods, chemistry books, obsessive concern for food, or, in most cases, nutritional supplements.

The suggestions I give in this book have worked for the thousands of women I have advised; they can work for you to restore the health and vitality you may have lost, from chronic dieting, following the chic low-fat, high-complex-carbohydrate diets, and fast-food eating. I offer a nutritionally sound program to put the right fats, red meat, eggs, whole grains, and even fast foods in their proper place in your diet, to eliminate mineral inhibitors such as sugar and caffeine, and to banish the fear of fat—forever. It is my hope that this book will help you learn by first-hand experience that health is not a matter of chance, but a matter of choice.

TWO

Nutrition Notes
for the Food-Wise Woman

Tell me what you eat and
I will tell you who you are

—Athelme Brillat-Savarin

Before You Begin

Are you nourishing your body for the challenges you face daily? Are you a chronic dieter like Susan, a nutrition buff like Pat, or a grabber like Maryann? Or even a combination of all three? One way to help you understand your patterns of eating and food choices is to keep a food diary, recording your total intake of food and beverages for a specified period of time.

At the end of this chapter, you will find three copies of a Food Diary Record Sheet for you to record your total food intake for three consecutive days. The Food Diary asks you to record not only the food eaten, but the method of preparation: broiled, grilled, or fried, for example. If there is a sauce or dressing, remember to record it.

Unless you usually measure your portions, estimate the amounts, to the best of your ability using standard measurements, e.g., ¼ cup or 4 ounces.

When you eat (Time of Day) is included since it may give you clues to patterns of overeating and will help you plan mealtimes and snacks. Where you eat (Setting) can be helpful to assess how frequently you eat at home, in restaurants, and in friends' homes, so you can better anticipate and plan for suitable food choices.

Finally, why you eat (Emotions) should be recorded so that you can begin to distinguish between true biological hunger and "emotional hunger." The role of emotions in stimulating and controlling our eating behavior is the focus of considerable research. For example, Janet Polivy, Ph.D., professor of psychology and psychiatry at the University of Toronto, has found that, when faced with stress or disappointment, women who diet are more likely to go off their diets and to eat more than women who aren't dieting. Emotional triggers are highly individual—some of us eat voraciously when we are in love; some of us take our anger out on a plate of pasta or share our joy with a hot fudge sundae. If you need to make changes in your eating patterns, noting these emotional triggers will be essential to success.

Include two workdays and one weekend day in keeping the food diary, to give you a more realistic picture of your overall pattern. Eat the way you ordinarily do, not the way you think you ought to for this record.

Once complete, your record becomes a valuable tool for putting the suggestions in this book to work. Look first at what you were eating and compare it against the following list of basics:

_____ One to two tablespoons of unprocessed oil a day (include salad dressings and cooking oils)

_____ Four or more servings of fruits and vegetables each day (a serving is ½ cup cooked or 1 cup raw)

_____ Three or more servings of complex carbohydrates from grains, starchy vegetables, and legumes (½ cup equals one portion)

_____ At least two 3-ounce portions of protein (lean beef, skinless poultry, seafood); 1 egg equals 1 ounce of protein (include up to 4 per week)

_____ At least two servings of a calcium source each day (such as 8 ounces of yogurt or milk, a large stalk of broccoli, or even a calcium supplement, if you are simply unable to consume dairy products or enough calcium from foods)

_____ A daily source of cholesterol-lowering soluble fiber, such as an apple, a sweet potato, or a cup of kidney beans

Next, make note of how many of the following calcium or iron inhibitors you find.

_____ Coffee

_____ Soft drinks

_____ Sugar

_____ Tea

_____ Chocolate

_____ Aluminum

Finally, review your food diary for the social and emotional patterns that affect your eating habits. Are any of the following true for you?

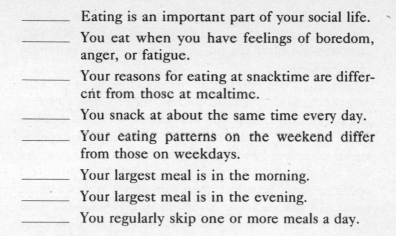

_____ Eating is an important part of your social life.

_____ You eat when you have feelings of boredom, anger, or fatigue.

_____ Your reasons for eating at snacktime are different from those at mealtime.

_____ You snack at about the same time every day.

_____ Your eating patterns on the weekend differ from those on weekdays.

_____ Your largest meal is in the morning.

_____ Your largest meal is in the evening.

_____ You regularly skip one or more meals a day.

When you read my program, you will learn how to apply this information to the insights from your food diary to design the optimum plan for yourself. You can make better food choices and substitute foods that will cover areas in which you are deficient.

If your reasons for eating include depression, anxiety, boredom, tension, or fatigue, then your eating style is being controlled by emotional triggers, rather than by hunger and nutritional need. Identifying these triggers is the first step in modifying your behavior.

If your social eating has an emotionally based component (a desire to be accepted or anxiety at new social settings) then anticipating these events can help you plan ahead for them. You will have a variety of choices for foods and beverages, all of which could enable you to fulfill any social needs without abandoning the plan. Chapter Eleven even has some suggestions for eating out within the plan.

Studies have shown that people who successfully changed their eating habits and food choices did so by making relatively modest changes in what, how much, and how often they ate. The less drastic the changes and the closer they matched the way the individuals normally ate and could eat in the future, the more successful these changes were.

So when you complete your review and begin your plan for change, be realistic and decide on small, concrete steps. For example, if you find that you are most apt to grab "junk food" in the midafternoon when hunger pangs strike, plan ahead and keep fresh fruit handy. If you find that you tend to skip breakfast and lunch, and overeat at dinner, make an effort to eat something in the morning and early afternoon—even a Spicer's Wheatsnack (see Chapter Ten) or a fruit shake. If fiber is your deficiency but you hate oat bran cereals, then get your fiber from beans or raw fruits or vegetables.

You will find that the menu plans and recipes in Chapter Twelve do not generally include exotic ingredients; in many cases, they represent a stepping-off point, a halfway measure to move you toward long-term health and well-being.

The Nutrition Notes

You have decided—you choose health. You want to feel better, look better, and live better now and in the future. This section summarizes my approach, developed through counseling thousands of women and described in greater detail in following chapters, to help you achieve this goal.

- Don't Be a Yo-Yo. The yo-yo diet syndrome (the lose, gain, and regain cycles) can be more hazardous to health than remaining overweight. Very low calorie diets, particularly when combined with exercise, can drastically lower metabolic rate. Chronic dieters can regain more fat faster with regained fat redistributed around the abdominal area, which increases the risk of diabetes and heart disease. The ratio of fat to lean protein also increases with constant dieting and the risk of heart disease can rise as much as 30 percent.

By putting essential fats in your diet and following the other notes outlined here, you will lose weight without crash dieting.

• Optimize calcium intake. As I stress in Chapter Eight, choose high-quality calcium foods. Nonfat dairy products, including yogurts, dry curd cottage cheese, and the new part-skim-milk Lifetime cheeses, are among the most concentrated calcium sources. You can get calcium from other sources as well, especially if you are allergic to dairy products. These include green, leafy vegetables like broccoli, bok choy, kale, and collard greens. Sea vegetables like hijiki (popular in Japanese cuisine) contain 14 times the calcium of a glass of milk. Wakame provides 1,300 milligrams calcium in a little less than ½ cup, while kombu provides 800 milligrams in the same sized portion.

Take full advantage of the calcium you do get by eliminating the inhibitors: soft drinks, cocoa, coffee, tea, aluminum, and excessive grain intake. Remember, the phosphoric acid in soft drinks (regular and diet), the phytic acid in grains, and the caffeine in chocolate, coffee, and tea all interfere with calcium absorption or increase its excretion. Aluminum from pots and pans, cans, antacids, baking powders, and even tap water leach calcium from your body.

• Perform Weight-Bearing Exercises. Research has shown that such exercise helps retain calcium in your bones. If you want to burn fat in the process, try to maintain continuous movement for 45–60 minutes daily. Brisk walking, cycling, rowing, swimming, or rebounding on a mini-trampoline are the best exercises to burn fat calories. Activities like calisthenics, volleyball, racquetball, and tennis, which feature stop and start movements, are best to burn carbohydrates. The most efficient fat burning occurs when you exercise before a meal, not after.

- Beef Up Blood-Building Iron. Consume at least two servings (3 ounces each) of lean beef weekly and include iron-rich legumes and green, leafy vegetables in your diet. Vegetarians should emphasize iron-rich beets and can consider herbal supplements like yellow dock and dandelion root for easily assimilable iron. A high vitamin C source, like citrus fruits, tomatoes, or a baked potato, eaten with the iron-rich food further enhances iron absorption. Cooking in cast-iron pots contributes small amounts of vital iron to foods.

- Include Eggs and Beef. There are other reasons, besides your need for extra iron, to include beef in your regular diet, as I discuss in Chapter Four. It is a valuable source of zinc; the stearic acid it contains may actually lower serum cholesterol levels. Eggs contain the richest source of the sulfur-bearing amino acid l-cysteine, so important for skin, hair, and nail health. Both foods are low-calorie, economical sources of protein, manganese, and other essential minerals. At least 4 eggs, including those used in baking, and 2 three-ounce servings of red meat weekly are recommended in my plan.

- Put Fats in Their Place. Include two tablespoons of essential fat every day in salad dressings and cooking.

Restrict your total fat intake to an average of 20–30 percent of total daily calories. This means that the average woman consuming a typical 2,000-calorie diet can have about 9 teaspoons of fat from all sources per day, equal to 44 grams of fat. Women should generally opt for between 40 and 50 grams of fat daily.

Eliminate all sources of damaged fats, such as commercial vegetable oils, hydrogenated oil products (margarine and vegetable shortening), and all products containing them. Use only purified, unrefined, expeller-pressed raw or virgin oils.

Unless you are among the 10 percent who have diagnosed problems with high cholesterol levels (total cholesterol level above 200 milligrams, for example), you should not need to pay special attention to cholesterol if you are eating essential fats and following the other recommendations.

- **Control Your Sweet Tooth.** Avoid simple sugars, sweeteners, and refined carbohydrates. Keep your fruit consumption to three to five portions a day, preferably the fruit itself rather than juice. A portion is: 1 small banana, 12 cherries, 1 small apple, or ½ grapefruit; for more details, see Chapter Ten. Both refined sugar and natural sugar products (even fruit and fruit juice) can play havoc with your energy levels and contribute to high blood lipid levels of triglycerides. Sugar can cut calcium absorption and encourage yeast overgrowth, contributing to fatigue and a variety of allergic and mental symptoms. Excess sugar can also block the manufacture of beneficial prostaglandins from essential fatty acids.

- **Vary Complex Carbohydrates.** Choose more legumes and vegetables such as potatoes, squash, peas, and root vegetables. By diversifying your diet, you avoid gluten intolerance from overdoing consumption of grains like wheat, rye, oats, and barley; the phytic acid that inhibits calcium absorption; and the excess carbohydrates that may feed yeast infections.

- Value Vegetables Daily and Weekly. Vegetables contribute fiber, vitamins, and minerals for all-around health and should be part of your diet. Feature cruciferous vegetables like brussels sprouts, cabbage, broccoli, cauliflower, rutabagas, and turnips, at least twice a week, to help reduce the risk of cancer. Eat dark green, yellow, or orange vegetables at least 3–4 times per week for their rich beta carotene content. Vegetables high in beta carotene protect cells from environmental damage, keep skin in top shape, and carry cancer protection.

- Fiber Up Your Diet. Americans eat approximately 10–20 grams of fiber per day, yet the National Cancer Institute suggests between 25 and 35 grams to help prevent colon and rectal cancer. Choose a balance of water-soluble fibers from oats, legumes, sweet potatoes, and other fresh fruits and vegetables to control cholesterol and even out blood sugar levels.

- Avoid Too Much Salt. Excess salt contributes to high blood pressure and fluid retention and bloating. Many canned, frozen, bottled, and packaged foods contain hidden salt, so become a label reader. Avoid soy sauce, tamari, and salt added to foods at the table. Aim for an average daily intake of 1,500 milligrams, the equivalent of ¾ teaspoon. Remember that many foods are naturally high in sodium, including carrots, celery, and beets. Eating a well-balanced diet, without ever using a salt shaker, will give you all the sodium you need for good health.

- Cook for Health. Choose healthy cooking methods for your healthy foods. Baking, roasting, broiling, poaching, and steaming are best for daily cooking. Frying, charcoal grilling, and smoking should be limited because of the harmful chemicals they produce in food.

- Avoid Aluminum. Do not use aluminum or foil for cooking, reheating, or wrapping foods. This pliable heavy metal leaches into acidic foods and deposits in the kidneys, brain, and intestines. It has been associated with Alzheimer's disease and interferes with the body's ability to absorb and process calcium through chemical interaction with other minerals.

FOOD DIARY

Day of the week _____

What (Name of food/ preparation)	Amount (Portion size)	When (Time of day)	Where (Setting)	Why (Emotions)
Meal one				
Meal two				
Meal three				
Snacks				

FOOD DIARY

Day of the week _____

What (Name of food/ preparation)	Amount (Portion size)	When (Time of day)	Where (Setting)	Why (Emotions)
Meal one				
Meal two				
Meal three				
Snacks				

FOOD DIARY

Day of the week _____

What (Name of food/ preparation)	Amount (Portion size)	When (Time of day)	Where (Setting)	Why (Emotions)
Meal one				
Meal two				
Meal three				
Snacks				

THREE

The Case Against Fat-Free,
High-Grain Diets

*The American diet has become dangerous
in many more ways than one.*

—Adelle Davis, nutritionist

There are many health-conscious women like Pat and Gina who are still following the standard dietary model of the 1970s and 1980s—a no-fat, high-complex-carbohydrate diet. What they need to understand is that their fat-free, predominantly grain-based foods may actually be creating many of the health problems women face in the 1990s. Women are eating their way into hormonal dysfunction.

In 1974, when Nathan Pritikin published his book, *Live Longer Now,* he struck a responsive chord for many Americans. The American Heart Association was urging us to cut back on fat consumption, and the death rate from cardiovascular disease was continuing its steady rise.

Although he was not a physician, Pritikin had reviewed countless pieces of research over a 25-year period.

31

When he was diagnosed in 1955 with a severe heart condition, he began reviewing medical literature on the degenerative diseases of the Western world such as cardiovascular disease, high blood pressure, diabetes, and cancer. He came to the landmark conclusion that the fat in our diet was the culprit. He believed that by severely reducing our fat intake to just 5–10 percent of calories and increasing complex carbohydrates to 80 percent, we could achieve the lower rates of degenerative diseases seen in native cultures like the Bantus of South Africa and the Tarahumara Indians of Mexico.

This was a spartan diet and Pritikin was criticized by the American Heart Association, the American Diabetes Association, and many physicians. Yet he persisted. He established the Pritikin Longevity Centers in California, Florida, and Pennsylvania. Today, a few years after his death in 1985, most experts and professional organizations all over the country have moved toward his recommendations, including many of those who had previously criticized him.

Concern over No-Fat

Something was not quite right, however. The Pritikin diet and others like it did not prove to be the miracle we sought. I saw it in the participants I worked with as nutrition director of the Pritikin Longevity Center in Santa Monica and later in private practice: women who should have felt good and looked good on their low-fat, high-carbohydrate diet were instead tired, cold, retaining fluids, and experiencing menstrual difficulties and recurring yeast infections. Their diet records revealed they were hungry most of the time and tried to raise their energy levels with sugar-laden cookies, fruit juices, and frozen yogurt. Their hair and skin were dry, their nails brittle and ridged. Many had stopped menstruating.

The factor of the ridged nails, which I recounted in my first book, *Beyond Pritikin*, has created quite a stir among my readers. I have received countless letters from readers all over the country who report their nails have developed ridges after being on a low-fat, high-complex-carbohydrate diet for several months. As I explained in *Beyond Pritikin*, this condition is a sign of a vitamin or mineral deficiency, which may be due to the high levels of fiber that take essential minerals like calcium and iron out of the body. Any diet that is not good for the hair, skin, and nails is not good for the rest of your body either.

Other experts also had doubts. If fats were the answer to Americans' high rate of degenerative diseases, how were the researchers to explain:

- The Eskimos, who despite a diet that is 70 percent fat, are free of cardiovascular disease.

- The Greeks and Italians along the Mediterranean, with a death rate from heart disease half that of Americans, yet with a diet of 40 percent fat (the typical American diet).

- The Masai tribe of East Africa, living on a diet comprised almost entirely of meat and milk, who show low blood cholesterol levels and negligible heart disease.

- The results of an 11-year study of residents of Roseto, Pennsylvania, who consume high-cholesterol and high-fat foods, which showed blood cholesterol levels averaging 224 (average for the nation) and almost no heart attacks in men under 55.

What we've learned is that fats are generally misunderstood and unduly maligned. Not only are some fats "good," but the essential fatty acids from the Omega 3s and 6s are vital to the integrity of the body's cell membranes and to the maintenance of the cardiovascular, immune, reproductive, and central nervous systems. These fats, along with their far-reaching health benefits, are the ones most likely to be deficient in a woman's diet.

How Fats Are Classified

Let's talk briefly about how fats are defined. All fatty acids are classified as saturated, monounsaturated, or polyunsaturated. (These terms relate to the type and number of hydrogen bonds in the chemical structure of the fatty acid.) Their structure affects the movement of the molecules and the susceptibility of the fat to heat and oxidation.

All fats are a blend of the three types, but one type predominates, giving the fat its status as a saturate, monounsaturate, or polyunsaturate. The chart below outlines the major food sources of each fat group:

Saturates *Animal sources:* pork, lamb, and beef fats (lard, tallow, suet); organ meats; full-fat dairy products such as whole milk, cream cheese, ice cream, and butter. *Vegetable sources:* coconut oil, cocoa butter, palm oil, and palm-kernel oil.

Monounsaturates *Vegetable, legume, and seed sources:* olive, avocado, almond, apricot kernel, peanut, canola (rapeseed), and high-oleic safflower and sunflower oils.

Polyunsaturates (Omega 3) *Animal sources:* marine oils from salmon, mackerel, herring, cod, sardines, rainbow trout, shrimp, oysters, halibut, tuna, sablefish, bass, flounder, and anchovies; cold-water fish such as trout and crappie. *Vegetable sources:* flax (linseed) oil, pumpkin seed, canola, soybeans, walnuts, wheat germ, wheat sprouts, fresh sea vegetables, leafy greens.

Polyunsaturates (Omega 6) *Animal sources:* mother's milk, organ meats, lean meats. *Vegetable sources:* safflower, sunflower, corn, soy, cottonseed, sesame, raw nuts and seeds, legumes, spirulina, leafy greens. *Botanicals:* borage, evening primrose oil, and gooseberry oil.

Percent of Fatty Acids by Saturation Type in Various Oils

Type of Oil	Saturated	Mono-unsaturated	Poly-unsaturated
Almond	9	65	26
Apricot kernel	6	63	31
Avocado	20	70	10
Canola	6	60	34
Coconut	92	6	2
Corn	17	29	54
High-oleic safflower*	8	75	17
High-oleic sunflower*	8	81	11
Olive	10	82	8
Palm kernel	83	16	1
Peanut	13	60	27

Type of Oil	Saturated	Mono-unsaturated	Poly-unsaturated
Safflower	8	13	79
Sesame	13	46	41
Soy	14	28	58
Sunflower	8	26	66

Source: Adapted from Spectrum Naturals, Petaluma, CA.

*High-oleic oils are produced from a new breed of sunflower and safflower seed, which contains higher levels of the mono-unsaturated fatty acid, oleic acid.

Saturated Fats

Saturated fats are the current "bad guys" in the American diet because they have been connected with high cholesterol and hardening of the arteries. The real problem is that they are often eaten in excess. Furthermore, they are found in many of our most popular foods, like full-fat dairy products such as cheese and ice cream, as well as tropical vegetable oils such as palm, palm kernel, and coconut oils used in many baked goods. Cookies, candies, cakes, crackers, and cereals often contain one or more of these highly saturated vegetable oils. Although many manufacturers are now removing palm and coconut oil from their products, they are substituting 100 percent vegetable shortening. Hydrogenated fats like vegetable shortening and margarine function the same way saturated fats do in the body and are not healthy substitutes.

The good news is that meat is healthier than previously believed. A recent study in the *New England Journal of Medicine* suggests that the stearic acid component in beef fat may be helpful in lowering cholesterol and in moderating other fats in the diet. So if you are concerned about saturated fats, you do not have to eliminate red meat completely—simply choose lean cuts such as the tip or eye of the round and top round, which rate close to chicken in levels of fats and calories but contain more minerals.

Monounsaturated Fats

There is now an all-purpose monounsaturated vegetable oil on the market called canola oil. Similar in composition to olive oil (60 percent monounsaturates versus 82 percent in olive), "canola" means Canadian oil. It is a result of special plant breeding from the rapeseed, a member of the mustard seed family. Canola is one of the lowest of all oils in saturated fats and is one of the few vegetable sources of Omega 3s.

Research by Scott M. Grundy, M.D., director of the University of Texas Health Sciences Center, has highlighted the special benefit of monounsaturated fats. In the *New England Journal of Medicine*, March 1986, Dr. Grundy reported that monounsaturates lowered total blood cholesterol levels even more than a low-fat, high-carbohydrate diet did. Perhaps more important, the monounsaturate high-oleic safflower oil selectively lowered the "bad' cholesterol and left more of the "good" cholesterol than did the polyunsaturate safflower oil (more about cholesterol in Chapter Four).

Polyunsaturated Fats: The Essential Fatty Acids

There are 45 essential nutrients that are critical for total body function. These include 20 minerals, 15 vitamins, 8 amino acids (the building blocks of protein), and 2 fatty acids (the building blocks of fat). These nutrients cannot be made from other substances; we must get them in the natural state from foods or, in some cases, dietary supplements.

We need a balance of the proper essential fats from both the Omega 3s and 6s. These two groups of polyunsaturated fatty acids are essential for the regulation of every function in the human body. From the original Omega 3 fatty acid, alpha-linolenic acid, our bodies make eicosapentaenoic acid (EPA) and docosahexaenoic acid (DHA). From the original Omega 6 fatty acid, linoleic, our bodies produce gamma-linoleic acid (GLA). These two series of essential fatty acids are found naturally in Omega 3–rich cold-water fish and unprocessed Omega 6–rich vegetable, seed, and botanical oils. Both groups must be provided by the diet because the body cannot produce them itself.

Once known as vitamin F, these essential fatty acids (EFAs) must be present in the diet along with vitamin E and the B vitamins to produce sex and adrenal hormones and control cell growth. The benefits credited to polyunsaturates are actually the health benefits provided by the essential fatty acids or EFAs.

For example, the EFAs are a component of the outer membrane of every cell, where they protect against invading viruses, bacteria, and allergens. Flexibility and fluidity of the cell membrane depend on the presence of the EFAs. EFAs increase metabolism and energy production. They help dissolve body fat into body fluids (yes, fat to lose fat!), decreasing blood cholesterol and triglyceride levels. They distribute the fat-soluble vitamins A, D, E, and K throughout the body, insulate the nerves, and help maintain equal body temperature.

Essential fatty acids are also the building blocks from which prostaglandins are made. These hormonelike substances regulate every organ, tissue, and cell in the human body at a basic cellular level.

Research continues on the exact roles of the three main types of prostaglandins and their many subgroups. What is known, however, is that they strengthen immunity, regulate sodium excretion, stimulate hormone production, contract intestinal muscles, and regulate blood clotting. One type stimulates production of thyroid hormone, assuring the energy we need. Prostaglandins also block your body's production of histamine, the chemical responsible for the itching eyes, stuffy nose, and scratchy throat in an allergic reaction. Decreased levels of prostaglandins may bring on some types of asthma; researchers know that if levels are adequate, muscles in the lungs relax and blood flow increases. Prostaglandins have proven helpful in relieving various premenstrual syndrome (PMS) symptoms as well as depression and conditions ranging from arthritis and ulcers to migraines and cancer.

The specific essential fatty acids needed for prostaglandin production are alpha-linolenic acid and cis-linoleic acid. In brief, the process is:

1. Alpha-linolenic acid (from the Omega 3 family of fatty acids) is converted to eicosapentaenoic acid (EPA). Helping with this conversion are vitamin B_6, magnesium, zinc, insulin, and an enzyme.

2. EPA is converted to the prostaglandin E_3 (PGE_3).

The chemical conversion process for the Omega 6 fatty acid, cis-linoleic acid, is very similar:

1. Cis-linoleic acid is converted to gamma-linoleic acid (GLA), again with the help of vitamin B_6, magnesium, zinc, insulin, and an enzyme.

2. GLA undergoes a chemical change to produce prostaglandin E_1 (PGE_1), aided by vitamins B_3 and C.

3. Alternatively, GLA can be converted to arachidonic acid through the action of another enzyme.

4. Arachidonic acid is then converted to prostaglandin E_2 (PGE$_2$).

The best sources of cis-linoleic acid are oils that are 100 percent expeller-pressed and unrefined. These oils are produced, not with solvents or chemicals, but by pressing the cooked raw material (sesame seeds, olives, etc.) through a screw press at the lowest possible temperature to release the oils. Unlike refined oils, an unrefined oil is not filtered a second time, bleached, or deodorized; it retains more of the nutrients of the source material.

Since cis-linoleic acid is converted to GLA before its ultimate production of prostaglandins, you can also sustain this process by using some of the plants and oils that contain GLA itself: borage, spirulina (a type of plankton), evening primrose oil, and gooseberry oil.

The Omega 3 alpha-linolenic acid is found in wheat sprouts, wheat germ, nuts and seeds (and their oils) including walnuts, flaxseeds, and soybeans. The direct form of EPA is found in high amounts in cold-water fish oils from fatty fish such as sardines, salmon, and mackerel. It is more potent in the fresh varieties and can deteriorate quickly in the freezing or canning process.

Commercially processed oils, hydrogenated margarines, and fried foods—what I call damaged fats—interfere with the transformation of GLA and EPA into prostaglandins. The once-beneficial polyunsaturates have been exposed to processing in the form of excess heat, air, light, or hydrogenation that makes them now unusable for the human body. Without the ability to transform into prostaglandins, the EFAs are biologically worthless.

There are several other factors that hamper prostaglandin production by blocking the enzyme that transforms cis-linoleic acid into GLA. These factors include saturated fats, cholesterol, aging, alcohol, high blood sugar, viral infection, radiation, and aspirin. Thus, many individuals may have difficulty in obtaining the proper expeller-pressed unrefined oils in the first place, while others have difficulty in converting EFAs into prostaglandins because of dietary, illness, medication, and lifestyle factors.

The Fat–Weight Loss Connection

Eating the right fat will also help you achieve balanced weight loss. GLA has been found to stimulate the brown fat of the body. Thanks to the research of Dr. George Bray, the leading American expert on brown fat, we now know that brown fat is a special fat-burning tissue that burns and dissipates excess calories for heat, rather than depositing them for storage as fat. Unlike white fat, which is the insulating layer on the outside of the body, brown fat lies deeper, surrounding organs such as the heart, kidneys, and adrenals. Researchers have hypothesized that thin people may have activated brown fat, while overweight individuals may have dormant brown fat. It takes a certain type of fat to activate the brown fat. GLA, one of the EFAs we have been discussing, found directly in borage and evening primrose oil or in the preliminary form in safflower oil, stimulates brown fat metabolism.

I've had numerous case histories of women who were not able to lose weight until oil was added back into (not subtracted from) their diets. One such woman I met recently was a free-lance writer for a large newspaper who interviewed me on *Beyond Pritikin*. She was so taken in by the anti-fat propaganda that I made her a bet that she would lose at least one to two pounds a week if she added at least one to two tablespoons of unprocessed, unheated oil into her diet. I pointed out some of the tasty salad dressing recipes from the book. She particularly liked the sound of the Safflower Dressing with Papaya and Tarragon, and so agreed to add it to her salads twice a day. She called me one week later, delighted that she had lost not one pound, but three and one-half pounds on her diet with no change in her food intake, except for the oil.

The Fat-Yeast Connection

Essential fatty acids, especially in the Omega 3 group, slow down the progress of yeast organisms in the body. Yeast overgrowth is thought to affect as many as one in three Americans. Overgrowth of *Candida albicans*, common in women, causes symptoms ranging from allergies to throat infections to joint swelling to memory loss, and repeated vaginal or bladder infections. The EFAs stimulate the process of oxidation, which spells death to the oxygen-hating (anaerobic) yeast.

Healthy skin, hair, and nails owe much to the EFAs. EFAs plump up the cell membranes and help repair old membranes and construct new ones. Eczema, psoriasis, dandruff, hair loss, dryness, and brittle nails respond to added EFAs in the diet. The resurgence in popularity in the late 1980s of the liquid protein diets or fasts has been accompanied by a resurgence in one of its side effects: significant hair loss has resulted from the lack of EFAs in the formula.

By helping to control the flow of body oils, EFAs regulate the skin's metabolism and counter thick, dry skin from the inside out. Healthy collagen is also a benefit from the EFAs. The beautifying skin vitamins A and E must be dissolved in fat to be used within the body to provide glowing skin and hair.

Carrying vitamin D as well as calcium into the soft tissues, EFAs help protect against osteoporosis since calcium must have vitamin D present for absorption. Depletion of calcium from bones leads to brittleness.

Concern over High Carbohydrates

A low-fat, high-carbohydrate diet causes problems because it doesn't include adequate essential fat, but it causes an equal number of problems by emphasizing carbohydrates, in the form of excessive grains.

The popularity of low-fat, high-carbohydrate diets is just one factor in the phenomenal rise in grain consumption over the past 15 years, especially wheat, which represents over 80 percent of our total grain consumption. Wheat consumption has risen from 137 pounds per person in 1972 to 163 pounds today.

Beatrice Trum Hunter, food editor of *Consumers' Research Magazine* and author of *Gluten Intolerance*, has found that:

- Present-day food technology relies heavily on wheat—as emulsifiers, stabilizers, and food starches in such varied foods as ice cream, catsup, and some instant coffees.

- The growth of vegetarianism spurred many new ways to serve grains.

- The "gentrification" of pasta changed it from a food for the poor or a food that was considered "fattening," to a gourmet food item capable of being "dressed up or down."

- Urged to increase fiber intake, we have expanded our consumption of cereals, meals, and flours.

- Interest in ethnic cuisines, many of which include more grains than does standard American fare, has also played a part.

Grains are relative newcomers in the human diet—it has been only about 10,000 years since the development of agriculture. As a 1985 article in the *New England Journal of Medicine* points out, our prehistoric ancestors ate raw vegetables and low-fat meats with occasional seasonal fruits and nuts and seeds. They did not eat grains or dairy products.

Our digestive system has changed very little since then, but our diets have changed significantly.

Women, in particular, are learning that excesses of even the "best" food, including carbohydrates, can cause health problems. Many of these problems with carbohydrates actually stem from an ingredient of many grains, called gluten. Gluten consists of the two protein substances, glutenin and gliadin. Gliadin seems to be the problem in sensitive individuals.

Symptoms of gluten intolerance (also known as celiac disease, sprue, or gluten-induced enteropathy) were described almost 2,000 years ago. Once rare, these symptoms are now increasing. They include diarrhea, anemia, muscle spasms and cramps, bone or joint pain, headache, bloating, and intestinal pain.

There appears to be a genetic predisposition, but diet is the initiating factor. The gluten damages the intestinal lining, which then does not properly absorb the products of digestion. Minerals, vitamins, proteins, and fats pass out of the body, unused. Loss of vitamin D, calcium, and phosphorus brings on bone changes and muscle cramps. Loss of vitamin B_{12} and folic acid may bring on pernicious anemia; loss of iron can create iron deficiency anemia.

The high fiber content of gluten-rich grains (wheat, rye, oats, and barley), taken in excess, can help remove valuable nutrients such as zinc, calcium, and iron from the body before they can be absorbed and used. Both zinc and calcium are necessary for the release of insulin from the pancreas to metabolize sugar and other carbohydrates.

Phytates

Women may find they develop calcium deficiencies on a high-carbohydrate diet for another reason. Grains, particularly wheat, rye, and oats, unless they are sprouted, contain phytic acid, a phosphorus-like compound that interferes with calcium absorption. Phytic acid is primarily found in the husk of the grain, so there are high levels in bran. Many unsuspecting health-conscious people are washing away their calcium with daily doses of wheat or oat bran. Phytic acid also affects iron, magnesium, and zinc absorption. Mineral malabsorption is rampant these days, as evidenced by the rise in osteoporosis and increase in bone spurs, all signs of inadequate calcium metabolism.

The popularity of commercially yeasted breads may also be contributing to mineral problems. Yeast in breads does not remove the phytic acid from dough the way natural leavening, or sourdough, can. The natural fermentation process produces an enzyme that neutralizes the phytic acid. Furthermore, the longer natural leavening process breaks down the outer husks of the grain to release naturally contained minerals into the dough for greater availability to the body.

(An added advantage to naturally leavened, or sour-dough, bread is its sweet taste and moist texture, kept fresh longer by a crisp crust.)

What This Book Offers

The Supernutrition for Women Program includes essential and healthy oils, from food sources such as dark deep-sea fish and from oils such as safflower, sesame, olive, or canola. It avoids the saturated fats from full-fat cheeses and ice cream and hydrogenated fats from commercial vegetable oils, margarine, and shortening that have been associated with disease and aging.

I emphasize variety, ensuring consumption of a wide range of vegetables, fruits, protein, nonfat milk, and complex carbohydrates. This means putting lean meat and eggs back into your diet; it means using all the available sources of calcium, like green leafy vegetables, not just full-fat dairy products. Variety will give your body maximum exposure to all the essential nutrients from food sources without risking the problems of excesses— gluten intolerance, yeast infections, and degenerative diseases.

With the recommended food plan, you get the fiber you need without the gluten you don't need. Rice, fruit, vegetables, and beans offer high-fiber alternatives.

You will learn not only what to include but also what to avoid. My program makes a quantum leap from the dietary model of the 1970s and 1980s to nutrition in the 1990s with essential fatty acids, a cornerstone for health, beauty, and immunity.

FOUR

Why Women Need Meat and Eggs

The human organism needs an ample supply of good building material to repair the effects of daily wear and tear.

—Indra Devi, yoga teacher and writer

The egg—a natural, unprocessed food. Within its shell, it has every vitamin except C; it is the best dietary source of the sulfur-bearing amino acid, l-cysteine, so essential for healthy nails and skin and lustrous hair. It is an important source of trace minerals such as selenium. Its protein comes closest to matching the protein pattern best used by the body (so more of its protein's amino acids are put to use).

So why are all the beauty-conscious women who come to see me avoiding eggs? Why are women choosing bran muffins or processed cereals over omelets for breakfast? Why did the U.S.D.A. find egg consumption by women dropped 24 percent between 1977 and 1986? And what are the consequences of these choices to women like Susan, the chronic dieter; Pat, the nutrition buff; and Maryann, the grabber, described in Chapter One, all of whom seldom eat eggs?

47

There is a disturbing trend among women who are choosing not to eat meat, especially beef. Many women proudly assert that they don't eat any red meat at all. On the other hand, their diet histories reveal full-fat cheeses, cheese spreads, gourmet ice cream, and fast-food fish sandwiches—all higher sources of dietary fat than the red meat they avoid.

Although average consumption of fish and poultry has remained almost constant between 1977 and 1986, beef consumption among women has dropped 43 percent. Can we afford to give up such an excellent source of iron, vitamins B_2 (niacin), B_{12}, and riboflavin, and zinc? Our cold, tired bodies may be giving us the answer.

What appears to be the major factor in these dietary changes is the 30-year-long crusade against cholesterol, a crusade that many experts now believe is based on faulty logic and misunderstandings about cholesterol in the diet versus cholesterol in the bloodstream.

The Basics of Cholesterol: How It Works

I know you may have heard this before, but it bears repeating. Cholesterol is a waxy, fatlike substance found in foods of animal origin, such as beef, poultry, and eggs. To make sure you are adequately supplied, your liver and brain manufacture about 80 percent of the cholesterol found in your body.

Cholesterol is essential to good health. It is considered so vital that it is contained in practically every cell of the body and aids in cell membrane repair. Cholesterol in the skin reacts to sunshine to produce vitamin D. Much of the brain is composed of cholesterol, and it forms the insulation around nerve fibers. Cholesterol is necessary for the production of cortisone, an adrenal hormone in particular demand during physical stress.

Deficiencies of cholesterol have been associated with anemia, acute infection, and excess thyroid function. Significantly depressed cholesterol values have been found in patients with autoimmune disorders.

Cholesterol is not soluble in water, so to travel through the bloodstream, it is wrapped in water-soluble lipoproteins [lipids (fats and oils) + proteins]. These lipoproteins are categorized according to their protein content, or density. High-density lipoproteins (HDLs) carry excess cholesterol to the liver where it is broken down to bile acids and eventually flushed out of the body. For this reason, HDLs are referred to as "good" cholesterol. Low-density lipoproteins (LDLs) carry fats and cholesterol to the cells throughout the body, including the arteries, and deposit them for use.

Women under 50 tend to have higher levels of HDL than men do in the same age range; some experts believe this may be one factor in the lower heart attack rate among women of this age group. Kenneth H. Cooper, M.D., M.P.H., director of the Aerobics Center, Dallas, Texas, has analyzed a variety of longitudinal studies and his own research to provide guidelines for women's cholesterol levels (measured in milligrams per decaliter, mg/dl) as follows:

Cardiovascular Risk by Cholesterol and Lipid Levels

Age	Total cholesterol	LDL	HDL	Triglycerides	Total: HDL ratio
Low to Moderate Risk					
20–39	157–197	90–127	> 45	58–106	1.9–3.6
40–59	186–235	110–155	> 49	73–140	2.0–4.0
60+	205–252	126–175	> 50	82–146	2.0–4.8

Age	Total cholesterol	LDL	HDL	Triglycerides	Total: HDL ratio
		High Risk*			
20–39	198–220	128–149	< 45	107–146	3.7–4.2
40–59	236–259	156–181	< 49	141–190	4.1–4.9
60+	253–276	176–198	< 50	147–206	4.9–5.5

Source: Adapted from *Controlling Cholesterol,* by Kenneth H. Cooper (New York: Bantam Books, 1988), p. 53.

*Insufficient data to definitely say that HDLs in women in this range clearly mean a high risk; this is the best estimate of risk at this time.
> = more than; < = less than.

The evidence for the belief that high levels of dietary cholesterol raise blood cholesterol levels is not as overwhelming as some would have us believe. Studies from the University of California at Los Angeles, the University of Missouri, and others find no correlation between cholesterol in the diet and heart attack rates. In a yearlong Canadian study of both the Pritikin low-fat diet and the American Heart Association limited-fat diet, neither diet lowered blood cholesterol levels in patients with early vascular disease.

The present concern over cholesterol in the diet began with a Russian study in 1913 by a physiologist, Nikolai Anitschkov. He fed rabbits huge doses of cholesterol, and the cholesterol content of their blood rose dramatically by several hundred percent. This stress caused atherosclerosis, and cholesterol was found at the site of arterial damage.

Later research found that feeding rabbits pure, fresh cholesterol does not damage their arteries. However, if the cholesterol is exposed to oxygen prior to feeding, its unstable molecules produce toxic by-products. As Alan R. Gaby, M.D., Maryland-based practitioner and nutrition author, has pointed out, "Blood vessel damage can be produced by feeding animals even tiny amounts of these oxidation products. . . . Dietary cholesterol is apparently dangerous only to the extent that it becomes oxidized."[1]

According to a 1979 study by Dr. C. B. Taylor reported in the *American Journal of Clinical Nutrition*, oxidized cholesterol from food sources that are left out at room temperature or that are fried, smoked, cured (sausage), or aged (cheese) can be highly atherogenic (plaque-producing).[2] It is not pure cholesterol that creates artery-clogging plaque, but rather the toxic substances produced by the oxidation of cholesterol. Oxidized derivatives of cholesterol are unstable and decompose into free radicals, which damage blood vessel walls.

Any animal food that has been exposed to the ravages of oxygen for extended periods of time is likely to contain chemically altered cholesterol. Cooking eggs is a good example. Hard-boiled or fried eggs produce the highest serum cholesterol; scrambled or baked eggs produce less; soft-boiled produce the least.

(Balanced with the concern for cholesterol in cooked eggs is consideration of the flu-like illness caused by the bacteria *Salmonella enteritidis*, which has increased in incidence in recent years. Both the Food and Drug Administration and the U.S.D.A. have found the risk of contracting the illness to be extremely small, except in some high-risk groups: the elderly, the very young, pregnant women, and people with weakened immune systems or other serious illness. To lessen the risk for these high-risk groups, the government suggests throwing out any cracked raw eggs; avoiding uncooked dishes made with raw eggs like Caesar salad and steak tartare; cooking eggs thoroughly until both white and yolk are firm, which is likely to increase the level of cholesterol in the yolk; and storing eggs and egg dishes in the refrigerator.)

Many experts cite the Framingham study of thousands of individuals over a 14-year period as evidence in support of a low-cholesterol diet. Yet the study's director, William Kannel, M.D., has pointed out that there was "no discernable association between the amount of cholesterol in the diet and the level of cholesterol in the blood." Half the people who died of heart attacks in the study did not have high cholesterol levels.[3]

The Food and Nutrition Board of the National Research Council, in fact, takes the position that normal Americans will not reduce the risk of heart attack by going on a low-fat, low-cholesterol diet. Others would agree, including John Story, M.D., Purdue University; George Mann, M.D., Vanderbilt University; and Michael Oliver, president of the British Cardiac Society. Edward Ahrens, M.D., longtime cholesterol researcher at Rockefeller University, sums up the case well—to deny everyone red meat, eggs, and dairy products when only a minute fraction of the population has a problem with high cholesterol reduces the joy of life unnecessarily. And, I would add, subjects women to unnecessary nutritional deficiencies.

Dietary Elements That Do Influence Heart Disease

If dietary cholesterol is not the factor advertisers would have us believe, what is? Actually, not one, but several factors appear particularly influential.

It is interesting to note that within the past 100 years,

there has been a 350 percent increase in cardiovascular disease, but the cholesterol content of the American diet has remained about the same. *Both sugar and processed oil consumption, however, have risen considerably*—for example, we have increased the percentage of daily calories from sugar from 11 to 24 percent just since 1910.[4]

Saturated fats do raise blood cholesterol levels. According to John Lakosa, M.D., cardiologist and chairman of the American Heart Association nutrition committee, "Saturated fats are four times more likely to raise blood cholesterol levels than dietary cholesterol itself." The liver makes cholesterol from the saturated fats, whether or not you've consumed dietary cholesterol.

Strict vegetarians who substitute soybean products like tempeh or tofu for meat are still getting dietary fat, even though it is not animal fat or cholesterol. Soybeans, with 30 percent of their calories from fat, are the highest in fat of any of the legumes.

Sugar also appears to play a key role in both cholesterol and triglyceride levels. Triglyceride is the substance that fills fat cells and is thought by many to be even more important than cholesterol in heart disease. Triglycerides increase in your bloodstream when you eat excessive amounts of carbohydrates from sugars in refined products, such as white flour and white sugar, fruits and fruit juices, and alcohols.

Tests at Brookhaven National Laboratory found that patients on a high-sugar, low-fat diet had triglyceride levels two to five times greater than those on a low-sugar, high-fat diet. Ancel Keys, M.D., and coworkers found that when men ate simple sugars, their serum cholesterol levels were high. These levels went down when complex carbohydrates from fruits and vegetables replaced the simple sugars (see Chapter Five for more on sugar).[5]

On the other hand, vitamin C has been shown in

animals to lower blood cholesterol levels. Studies by Constance Spittle Leslie, M.D., of Pinderfields Hospital, England, have convinced her that atherosclerosis is a deficiency disease. She found that vitamin C removed cholesterol from the arteries of patients with atherosclerosis.

Animals studies have also shown vitamin B_6 deficiency to be associated with atherosclerosis. Monkeys given B_6 had their cholesterol levels lowered, even when they consumed high-cholesterol diets. When they were made deficient in B_6, they rapidly developed atherosclerosis.

Also associated with the risk of heart attack are smoking, obesity, and lack of exercise.

Shopping Smart

By shopping selectively, you can enjoy red meat without adding dangerous levels of saturated fats. Range-fed or grazed beef are lower in total fat than grain-fed, with the added benefit of no hormones or antibiotics (see the Staples Shopping List in Chapter Ten for more information).

Meats are graded for "quality" as determined by the U.S.D.A., although there is no law requiring that packaged meats carry a label with their grade. Grading reflects appearance, flavor, and tenderness, and appears on about 75 percent of fresh beef.

The three basic grades are Prime, Choice, and Select (previously known as Good). Select has the lowest fat content, Prime the highest. Select will usually be the least expensive, Prime the most expensive. Select cuts will give you the nutrients you want, without the fats that you don't want. Look especially for eye or tip of the round (with 29 percent of its calories from fat) or flank steak (34 percent) versus T-bone steak (41 percent).

Meat, Eggs, and Minerals

Only about 10 percent of the population has a problem with metabolizing cholesterol. For the majority of women, *avoiding* red meat and eggs carries its own set of nutritional hazards.

I fully agree with Annette Natow, Ph.D., R.D., professor of nutrition at Adelphi University, New York, who was quoted in *Prevention* magazine in 1986, "It's almost impossible for most women to get anywhere near the iron they need from their diets."[6] The recommended daily average for premenopausal women and adolescent girls is 15 milligrams, yet the average American diet yields 6 milligrams or less for every 1,000 calories consumed. Furthermore, the body absorbs only about 10 percent of the iron consumed. Paul Saltman, a biology professor at the University of California, San Diego, estimates that 30 to 35 percent of American women have low body stores of iron.

Beef contains two and one-half times the iron of chicken. This iron, known as heme iron, is three to five times more easily absorbed than the non-heme iron of vegetables. The iron from dark green leafy vegetables is less than 10 percent absorbed, from dried yeast, less than 5 percent, while the iron in red meats is 30 percent absorbed. In addition, eating meat with iron-rich vegetables increases the absorption of the vegetable iron.

Major Sources of Iron

Food	milligrams/serving
Meat, Poultry, Fish (3½ oz)	
Beef liver	8.8
Clams	6.1
Beef, lean	3.7
Shrimp	2.6
Lamb, lean	1.9
Poultry	1.5
Salmon	1.2
Beans and Lentils (1 cup)	
Limas, dry, cooked	5.6
Green split peas, cooked	4.2
Lentils, cooked	2.1
Vegetables (1 cup)	
Spinach, cooked	4.7
Peas, green, cooked	4.2
Beans, green, cooked	2.9
Fruits (1 cup)	
Prune juice	10.5
Raisins	5.6
Dates	5.3
Apricots, dried	5.1
Other	
Almonds (1 cup)	6.7
Dry yeast (1 oz)	4.6
Blackstrap molasses (1 tbsp)	3.2

Source: Nutritive Value of Foods (HG 72, U.S. Department of Agriculture).

Iron enables the body to maintain high energy levels by increasing the blood's oxygen-carrying capacity. It combines with protein and copper to make hemoglobin, which is the body's oxygen carrier. Tiredness and fatigue are the common signs of iron deficiency. Symptoms may come on slowly as the body depletes its stores of iron to make hemoglobin. These symptoms include weakness, headaches, tingling sensations in the hands and feet, exercise intolerance, sexual disinterest, irritability, depression, swelling of the tongue, pale lips and skin, lackluster hair, and brittle nails.

Efficient muscle function depends on sufficient iron reserves, as does a good mental attitude. Iron boosts the body's resistance to stress and disease, and helps ward off invading bacteria, viruses, and infections.

Researchers of the U.S.D.A. have found that women deficient in iron have an impaired ability to maintain body temperature in the cold. Other U.S.D.A. studies found that women who consumed well below the RDA of iron woke up more frequently during the night than when their iron consumption was adequate.

Women who exercise to lose weight have an additional problem. Without adequate iron, these women's bodies burn mainly carbohydrates, not fat, for fuel during exercise. Less oxygen is used that way, but so is less fat!

Heavy menstrual flow can result in further loss of iron. This cause of iron loss can often go undetected as women become used to their menstrual cycles. Signs of excessive iron loss are most prevalent in women whose periods last longer than five days, who need to wear double pads, or who pass large clots.

Pregnancy puts such stress on the body's iron reserves that most experts agree that even a balanced diet cannot provide adequate levels of iron, so daily supplements of 30–60 milligrams are regularly prescribed. Lactating women's needs are not considered to be more than those of other women; however, supplements are usually prescribed for two to three months following birth to restore the body's iron stores.

Even women who eat red meat may not be getting full benefit from the iron they consume. The level of iron actually absorbed by the body is affected by several substances:

- Oxalic acid in fruits such as raspberries and concord grapes; vegetables such as dandelion greens, rhubarb, sorrel, and spinach; and in chocolate and cocoa inhibit absorption of the iron from these sources.

- Phytic acid in cereal grains and in commercially yeasted breads impedes iron as well as calcium absorption.

- Tannic acid in tea (regular and peppermint) binds with iron and prevents it from entering the bloodstream. Drinking tea with your meals can decrease iron absorption by 50 percent. If you must drink tea, have it at least one hour before or after an iron-rich meal.

- The phosphates and carbonates in soft drinks inhibit iron absorption, as do the polyphenols in coffee.

- EDTA, a widely used food preservative, can reduce iron absorption by 50 percent.

- Calcium inhibits iron absorption as well. So leave at least two hours between the time you take supplements rich in these nutrients.

You can enhance your iron absorption further by eating vitamin C foods (tomatoes, potatoes, green peppers, dark green vegetables, citrus fruit, strawberries) just before or with your iron-rich foods. Cooking in iron pots, especially highly acid foods like tomatoes, can put additional iron into your food.

Meat and eggs are among the best sources of vitamin B_{12} (cobalamin), another element necessary to avoid anemia. Women of childbearing age are urged to get 2 micrograms a day, pregnant and lactating women need 3 micrograms. Other sources of this valuable element are brewer's yeast, milk, sardines, mackerel, oysters, beef liver, and clams.

(Although meat and eggs do not supply folic acid, this element is also needed to prevent anemia and to assure the full use of vitamin B_{12}. It can be found in spinach, broccoli, asparagus, wheat germ, liver, orange juice, dried beans, and brewer's yeast. The RDA for women of childbearing age is 180 micrograms.)

Pork and beef are also excellent sources of zinc, another mineral commonly deficient in a woman's diet. In fact, beef has three times the zinc of chicken.

Approximately 100 enzymes in a woman's body have zinc as one of their components. Zinc is essential for the synthesis of body protein, vitamin A metabolism, proper growth, healing of wounds and burns, and development of the sex organs. It promotes the removal of harmful carbon dioxide and is directly involved in the body's metabolism of carbohydrates and energy. It forms part of the insulin component secreted by the pancreas. Zinc helps to enhance digestion, protects the body in stressful conditions, and plays an important role in many major metabolic reactions.

Zinc deficiency has been associated with lowered immunity, decreased fertility, undeveloped sex organs, poor senses of taste and smell, stretch marks, and white spots on the fingernails. In addition, chronic tiredness, hair loss, dandruff, and slow healing of wounds have been related to lack of zinc.

As I mentioned at the beginning of this chapter, eggs are one of the best dietary sources of sulfur and its transport amino acid, l-cysteine. This amino acid helps build collagen in the skin and helps transport oxygen in the bloodstream. It is necessary for the proper utilization of vitamin B_6. Sulfur itself is beneficial to skin and hair health, which may account for its being called "the beauty mineral." High levels can be found in the horny layer of the skin keratin and in hair and nails.

Meat and egg are important sources of the following other vitamins and minerals:

- **phosphorus**—for healthy bones and teeth; formation of genetic material, cell membranes, and enzymes.
- **selenium**—antioxidant that prevents breakdown of body chemicals.
- **vitamin A**—aids in building and maintaining healthy hair, skin, and mucous membranes; needed for proper bone and teeth development.
- **vitamin B_1 (thiamin)**—converts carbohydrates to energy for cells; essential to a healthy nervous system.
- **vitamin B_2 (riboflavin)**—maintains healthy mucous membranes; releases energy from foods.
- **vitamin B_3 (niacin)**—facilitates energy production.
- **biotin**—aids in making fatty acids; necessary to release energy from carbohydrates consumed.

My plan includes up to 4 eggs a week, either prepared alone or as components of other dishes, and up to 2 servings (3 ounces each) of lean red meat. In Chapter Ten, I have listed a variety of alternatives.

Getting the vitamins and minerals that we need every day is not as easy as it might seem—despite the bounty of our supermarkets. Transporting, storing, and various levels of processing often transform foodstuffs from nutrient-rich to nutrient-empty. A diet that excludes meat, eggs, or even entire food categories is a diet that means trouble for women. And unless a woman has abnormally high levels of serum cholesterol, such a diet is unnecessary. The plan that I outline in this book restores not only the variety and balance missing from so many women's diets but also the health and well-being for which these women search.

FIVE

Why Women Don't

Need Sugar

*From disease I have learned much which life could never
have taught me in any other way.*

—Goethe

Thanks to the anti-fat crusades of government agencies
and other organizations, more and more Americans are concerned about the kinds and amounts of fats in their diet.

What we have forgotten in our zeal is that too much
sugar—primarily the simple sugars like white table sugar,
fruits, and fruit juices—can also make fat and cholesterol
in the body the way excess nonessential saturated fat
does. And it affects calcium balance in the body as well.

Do we monitor our sugar intake as we do our fat
consumption? The answer is a resounding, No! And it
may be more difficult than you think. Sales of gourmet
cookies, premium ice creams, and desserts laden with
both sugar and fat are at an all-time high. Sales of candy
in the United States were just under $11 billion in 1988,
up from about $10.3 billion in 1987, according to industry
analysts. Restaurants find an increasing demand for the

richest desserts on their menus. *Family Circle* magazine reports that their best-selling issues always feature some delectable-looking dessert on the cover—strawberry shortcake was a recent annual winner!

In fact, today you will probably eat 30 teaspoonfuls of sugar. Yes, even those of you who avoid desserts and no longer add sugar to your coffee will probably come close to consuming your weight in sugar each year.

That's because everything from cigarettes to french fries has sugar in it—added in processing or occurring naturally. Commercial brands like Hellmann's mayonnaise, Skippy peanut butter, Lipton Cup-a-Soup, Ritz crackers, and General Foods Cafe Vienna coffee all contain sugar!

Processors have discovered that sugar is not just for sweetening. Added to foods like catsup, it helps retain colors; added to baked goods, it ferments yeast and imparts a brown crust to breads and rolls; in soft drinks it adds body and texture; in chewing gum, pliability. Molasses and corn syrup may be added to a restaurant's hamburgers. Raw potato slices are often dipped in sugar water before being fried. Refined sugar, added to air-cured tobacco in the blending process, enhances both flavor and the burning quality of cigarettes.

How Sweet It Was

A preference for sweet taste begins early—newborns given increasingly sweet liquids increase their rate of sucking. At one time, this preference may have had an evolutionary benefit. Gary Beauchamp, a biopsychologist at the University of Pennsylvania, concludes that the sweet tooth enabled prehistoric humans to select ripe fruits and berries to eat. We have, of course, long since gone beyond this straightforward connection between good taste and good food.

Our involvement with sweeteners is not only physical, but emotional as well. Consider some of the synonyms for *sweet* found in *Webster's Collegiate Dictionary: agreeable, fragrant, dear, wholesome, fresh, fine.* Where would personal relationships be without "sweetheart," "sweet talk," "sugarpie," or "sugar daddy"? Where would we be without the "sweet smell of success,"and "sweetness and light"? Who would rather be a "sourpuss" than a "sweetiepie"?

Yet all is not sweetness and light with sugar. Longstanding problems with tooth decay have affected generations; although bacteria in the mouth metabolize a variety of sugars, the ability of sucrose to be converted by the bacteria into long complex molecules that adhere to teeth to form plaque makes it especially troublesome.

The negative health effects of our love affair with sugar are being found in a wide range of illnesses. Of particular concern to women are the connections between sugar and candidiasis (yeast infections), premenstrual syndrome (PMS), excess weight, and osteoporosis, as discussed in later chapters.

Sugar Basics

Misconceptions about sugar abound. A case in point is a client of mine, a very successful career woman based in New York City, who called me one day to report that she was completely off sugar. Knowing of her strong sweet tooth, I asked her how she did it. She said she had gone to a well-stocked health food store and found ice cream made from rice, apple- and pineapple-juice-sweetened cookies, and candies made from barley malt. "I'm not eating any sugar anymore!"

She had fallen into the trap that so many of us do. She had simply substituted certain forms of sugar for others, but she surely was still eating sugar, albeit from so-called natural sources. What she had not realized was that sugar is sugar is sugar and our bodies do not know the difference.

Like this client, when we say sugar, most of us mean refined white granulated sugar. However, there are at least a dozen other kinds, from a variety of sources:

- **glucose** (dextrose)—the main blood sugar in our bodies, our number one energy source; present in many fruits and in the starches of vegetables such as corn.

- **fructose**—fruit sugar from fruits, juices, and honey; commercial varieties now use corn as a base. It is twice as sweet as sucrose when added commercially to cold products and about the same sweetness as sucrose in baked goods. Because it is absorbed more slowly than sucrose, it does not raise the blood sugar level as dramatically, so it is a better sugar source for controlled diabetics.

- **sucrose**—made up of equal portions of glucose and fructose, this is the most abundant sugar in plants; refined, usually from sugar cane or beets, it has no nutrients. It is best known as table sugar.

- **maltose**—malt sugar, formed by the breakdown of starch.

- **lactose**—milk sugar; less sweet than sucrose.

- **raw sugar**—partially refined sucrose (dirt and plant debris remain, along with some trace minerals).

- **brown sugar**—table sugar with a molasses coating.

- **powdered sugar**—table sugar ground into fine crystals with a small amount of starch added to avoid caking.

- **molasses**—residue after crystals of sugar are removed from beet juice or sugar cane; contains a variety of sugars. Blackstrap molasses contains measurable amounts of trace minerals, including calcium and iron.

- **maple sugar**—sucrose made from boiling maple sap.

- **honey**—natural syrup made up of fructose, glucose, maltose, and sucrose; sweeter than sucrose, it can raise blood sugar levels higher than sucrose does. Its composition, quality, and taste vary, with clover honey generally having more iron than other varieties.

- **corn syrup**—derived from corn starch; made up of glucose and maltose.

- **high fructose corn syrup**—also made from corn starch, with the fructose content increased by enzymes; sweeter than sucrose. It is now used in almost all regular soft drinks.

- **sorbitol, mannitol, and xylitol**—synthetic products, sugar alcohols; all are more slowly absorbed than glucose and cause lower insulin responses than either glucose or sucrose. All three have laxative effects on sensitive individuals, however, and cannot be used in great quantity. When sorbitol is used to replace sugars in food products, the end result may contain even more calories because of the use of added fat needed to make the sorbitol more soluble.

These sugars share a number of characteristics:

1. They all provide four calories per gram.

2. Except for molasses, and maple syrup and honey to a lesser degree, they have no nutritional value. Whatever vitamins, minerals, and fiber that might have

been present in the natural state have been removed in processing.

Blackstrap molasses provides 14 percent of the RDA of calcium and 28 percent of iron in one tablespoon. Molasses, honey, and maple syrup help keep food fresher longer, so they work well as a refined sugar substitute in many recipes.

3. The negative effects seem to be the same no matter which sugar you consume.

Sugars are simple carbohydrates and are found in fruits, fruit juices, and sweeteners like white table sugar, molasses, honey, and maple syrup. Complex carbohydrates, which are chains of sugars plus protein, fats, vitamins, and minerals, are the preferred fuel for body energy. They are found in whole grains, vegetables, and beans. When complex carbohydrates are eaten, they are broken down into their simple sugars over a sustained period of time. This provides fuel and a steady release of energy.

When simple sugars and highly processed carbohydrates are eaten, they are broken down almost immediately—acting as an almost pure chemical. This rapidly releases sugar directly into the bloodstream, signaling various hormones and the pituitary gland to tell the pancreas to produce insulin. This rapid rise in the blood sugar level causes the pancreas to overreact—so much insulin is produced that the blood sugar level drops precipitously. The result is a quick burst of energy, followed by an equally fast fall in energy levels—what I call the peaks and valleys of energy. Constant stress on the clusters of special pancreatic cells, called the islets of Langerhans, to produce insulin after repeated consumption of sugary/processed foods causes these cells to become exhausted. When they no longer can produce adequate insulin levels, the result is the diagnosis of diabetes mellitus (mellitus comes from the Latin word for honey), commonly called diabetes.

According to a scientific study, there is one simple sugar that does *not* cause a rapid blood sugar or insulin rise. That is fructose, which provides a slower, more steady supply of blood sugar, making it the sweetener of choice for diabetics. Of all the sweetener sources that have been investigated, fructose has the slowest blood sugar rise.

In an attempt to provide a means of comparison of the effect of various foods on blood sugar levels, scientists at the University of Toronto have proposed the Glycemic Index. Applied to carbohydrates, including sugars, the Index, when fully developed, may help diabetics and others interested in controlling their blood sugar levels to plan their meals more effectively. In a 1988 report in *Diabetes Care*, David Perkins and his associates concluded that, when included in the diet, starchy foods with a relatively low score on the Glycemic Index were associated with reductions in LDL cholesterol ("bad") and triglyceride levels. Some of the food items in this category include legumes; pasta; grains such as barley, parboiled rice, and bulgur; and whole grain breads such as pumpernickel. Comparing several sugars, the researchers found the average glycemic response level for maltose to be five times greater and glucose four times greater than that of fructose.

In the process of being metabolized, refined sugars rob the body of valuable nutrients—chromium, manganese, cobalt, zinc, copper, and magnesium. These nutrients are taken from the body's mineral reserves, contributing to common deficiencies in men and women.

Another factor in the deficiencies is simply the numbers—Michael Jacobson of the Center for Science in the

Public Interest has summarized this point: "When you consume 20 percent of your calories from sugar, that means you have to get all of your nutrients from 80 percent of your food. It's unlikely that you're going to get them."

Sweet Fakes

Artificial sweeteners unfortunately pose their own problems. Both saccharin, a petroleum derivative, and aspartame, a combination of two naturally occurring amino acids, are referred to as "nonnutritive sweeteners," which means that they provide no calories. There are health risks associated with each of these artificial sweeteners.

A National Cancer Institute study found that certain people, primarily heavy artificial sweetener users, heavy users who smoke, and women who consume sugar substitutes or diet beverages at least twice a day, are at greater risk from the ill effects of these sweeteners than other groups.

Saccharin has been around since 1900, but its widespread use began in the late 1960s as a replacement for the banned cyclamates then in use as an artificial sweetener. In 1977 a Canadian study indicated that when pregnant rats were fed large doses of saccharin, their male offspring developed bladder cancer. As a result, the Canadians banned saccharin and the U.S. Congress ordered warning labels on all saccharin products, like Sweet 'N Low. The National Academy of Sciences in 1978 evaluated the evidence and concluded that saccharin was primarily a promoter of other cancer-causing agents, a cocarcinogen.

In the meantime, G. D. Searle developed aspartame,

a combination of two amino acids and methanol (wood alcohol). Closer to sugar in taste—actually 180 to 220 times sweeter than sugar—but without the aftertaste of saccharin, aspartame was an immediate success, replacing saccharin in diet soft drinks and other food items.

Few long-term studies of the effects of aspartame have been done. However, reports to the Food and Drug Administration and the Centers for Disease Control indicate that, as more people consume the substitute in large quantities, health may be affected. In some circumstances, individuals may be getting high levels of methanol; for example, it is estimated that on a hot day after exercise, an individual drinking three 12-ounce cans of diet cola could easily consume as much as eight times the Environmental Protection Agency's recommended limit for methanol consumption. The most common complaints are dizziness, disorientation, tunnel vision, ear buzzing, loss of equilibrium, numbing of hands and feet, inflammation of the pancreas, high blood pressure, eye hemorrhages, and seizures.

Artificial sweeteners can stimulate hunger or cause addictive allergies, just as sugar does. In other words, we get the disadvantages of sugar, along with the proven or suspected disadvantages of artificial sweeteners.

Sugar and Excess Weight

A four-ounce candy bar is equivalent in calories to eight average apples. Yet anyone who eats both the candy bar and the apples can tell you: the candy will not satisfy your appetite the way the apples will.

Sugar foods tend to pack a lot of calories into small packages, so you tend to eat more to feel full. Sugar also stimulates your appetite and, in many people, creates cravings.

Sugar, like damaged fats, may very well be our most dangerous source of excess calories. Absorbed quickly, unused sugar is carried to the cells where it is converted to saturated fats (the nonessential fatty acids) and cholesterol.

These non-EFAs compete with EFAs for an enzyme, D_6D, thus interfering with production of GLA and prostaglandins. As I have described, GLA activates the body's special fat-burning tissue (brown fat) that burns excess calories for heat.

Japanese researchers have found that eating fat and sugar at the same time can be more fattening than eating equivalent amounts at least an hour apart. A high-fat, high-sugar food—chocolates, French pastries, cream pies, for example—causes you to store fat more readily. Thus, chronic dieters like Susan, who reward themselves for being careful all day by eating high-fat, high-sugar gourmet ice cream, are sabotaging their efforts at weight loss.

Are You a Sugar Addict?

In her popular book *Lick the Sugar Habit,* my friend Nancy Appleton says about herself, "I was a sugarholic." After 40 years of doughnuts, ice cream sundaes, and candy, Nancy was facing her fifth bout of pneumonia; she regularly suffered headaches, canker sores, varicose veins, and a chronic cough. She cured herself by changing her life-style, including eliminating sugar and chocolate from her diet.

Nancy offers a short questionnaire to analyze your own level of sugar addiction. I've reprinted it below. Answering these questions about your eating habits honestly may help you better evaluate the role of sugar in your present diet, so you can determine what, if any, changes are needed to restore your good health.

A Sugar Questionnaire

	True	False
1. I don't eat refined sugar every day.	_____	_____
2. I can go for more than a day without eating some type of sugar-containing food.	_____	_____
3. I never have cravings for sugar, coffee, chocolate, peanut butter, or alcohol.	_____	_____
4. I've never hidden candy or other sweets in my home in order to find and eat them later.	_____	_____
5. I can stop after one piece of candy or one bite of pastry.	_____	_____
6. There are times when I have no sugar of any kind in my home.	_____	_____
7. I can go for three or more hours without eating and not experience the shakes, fatigue, perspiration, irritability, depression, or anxiety.	_____	_____
8. I can have candy and other sweets in my home and not eat them.	_____	_____
9. I don't eat something sweet after every meal.	_____	_____
10. I rarely drink coffee and eat doughnuts or sweet rolls for breakfast.	_____	_____

11. I can go for more than an hour after waking up in the morning without eating.   _____   _____

12. I can go from one day to the next without drinking a soft drink.   _____   _____

Source: From *Lick the Sugar Habit* by Nancy Appleton, Ph.D. (Avery Publishing Group, Inc.: Garden City Park, NY 11040).

Scoring: If you marked "False" more than four times, you are probably sugar-sensitive: allergic and addicted to it. If you checked four or fewer "False" answers, you may indeed have sugar under control in your life. Or you may be fooled by the processors, unaware of just how pervasive sugar is in our diets.

Breaking the Sugar Habit

The sad fact is that even those of us who consider ourselves nutritionally aware are probably getting far more sugar than we need or want. From postage stamps to paper cups to bran flakes to hamburger buns, sugar is part of the processing. We choose fruit juice over sodas, getting more nutrients but almost the same amount of sugar. We buy sugar-free gum, unaware that the sugar alcohols used to sweeten them contain the same calories as sugar.

Just a few of the nonfood items that contain sugar are adhesives, hair spray, lozenges, tapes, aspirin, breath sprays, ointments, talcums, and toothpaste.

It would take an entire book to list the food items that contain high levels of sugar. There are many hidden sources of sugar in natural and manufactured form. Here are just a few:

Hidden Sugar

Food	Serving Size	Sugar* (tsp./serving)
Lowfat yogurt, fruit	1 cup	13
Fruit drink/punch	12 ounces	12
Cranberry sauce	½ cup	11.7
Beets, pickled (Delmonte)	½ cup	9.9
Frozen yogurt	½ cup	7
Regular soda	12 ounces	6–9
Angel food cake	1/12 cake	6
Jell-O Pudding Snacks	4 ounces	6
Chocolate bar	1 ounce	5
Applesauce, sweetened	½ cup	4.3
Apricots, dried	4–6 halves	4
Raisins	¼ cup	4
Chocolate fudge	1½-in. square	4
Doughnut, plain	3-in. diameter	4
Frozen yogurt, low-fat	½ cup	4
Vanilla ice milk	½ cup	3.4
Vanilla ice cream	½ cup	3.1
Brownie	2x2x¾-in.	3
Orange juice	4 ounces	2.5
Applesauce, unsweetened	½ cup	2
Nature Valley granola bars	0.8 ounce	1.5
Chewing gum	1 stick	0.5

Source: The U.S. Department of Agriculture, the American Dietetic Association, and the Center for Science in the Public Interest, among others.

*Approximate level of all sugars, natural and manufactured.

Some breakfast cereals may even contain over 50 percent sugar, natural or added; even those that do not add marshmallows or sugar coating are high sugar sources. Post Raisin Bran, for example, has the equivalent of 53 percent sugar in one half cup, while Fruit and Fibre contains 46 percent sugar in a half-cup serving. High-fiber cereals may be merely providing sugar-coated bran. While much, if not all, of the sugar in these examples is naturally occurring from the raisins, malt, and grains, sugar is sugar when it comes to many of its health effects.

Awareness, then, becomes the number one factor in controlling your sugar habit.

- Read the label to find out if the food you eat contains sugar. Search for any of the *-ose* words (glucose, dextrose, sucrose, etc.). Sugar can be listed as corn sweetener, corn syrup, or just sweetener. Ingredients on labels by law are listed with the ingredient in greatest quantity shown first, the second highest listed second, and so forth.

- Make your own muffins, puddings, gelatins, sorbets, and fruit desserts, where you can control sugar content. Generally, you can cut down the amount of sugar in a recipe by one third to one half without affecting taste. Use unsweetened fruit juice, molasses, maple syrup, or honey as sweeteners (see recipes in Chapter Twelve).

- Substitute unsweetened fruit juice mixed half and half with mineral water or seltzer for regular or diet soft drinks or even 100 percent fruit juice.

- Use fresh fruit as snacks or desserts, but watch you don't go overboard. They are high in natural sugar, but do carry fiber, vitamins, and minerals as well.

- Don't use sweets as rewards—for yourself or your

family. More than any other food, sweets become entangled in our psychological and emotional lives: we celebrate with a cake, we console ourselves with Haagen-Dazs. Learn your own triggers and work at breaking the habit. The food diary technique has been especially helpful for many of my clients.

For more suggestions, see Chapter Twelve.

SIX

Carbohydrates: When Enough
Is Too Much—Part I

Most illnesses which befall man arise either from
bad food or from excessive eating of good food.

—Anonymous

Poor Pat. Like so many, she is a real nutrition devotee. She follows the current dietary model—the low-fat, high–complex-carbohydrate diet—and yet still feels tired, bloated, and fights off vaginal yeast infections. Could these problems be related to diet? You may not think so, but something is going on. Let's review the situation.

Carbohydrates—fruits, vegetables, whole grains, and beans—are a valuable source of vitamins and minerals, including vitamins A, B, and C, phosphorus, and folic acid. They are the only sources of dietary fiber. They contain the same calories per ounce as protein and less than half the calories of fat. Jane Brody, health columnist for the *New York Times*, points out that they "are the only food category *not* linked to any leading killer diseases."[1]

However, they have been linked to several health

77

problems in today's woman. Excess consumption of grains is associated with both gluten intolerance and candidiasis (yeast infections). Other carbohydrates, including simple (sugars) and complex (starches), are also associated with candidiasis. As Shirley S. Lorenzani, Ph.D., has written, "It is no coincidence that Candida overgrowth is the twentieth century disease and sugar is the twentieth century food."[2] By enthusiastically embracing either a high-carbohydrate diet or a junk-food diet, women have once again set themselves up for ill health and needless suffering.

Candidiasis and the Contemporary Woman

What are Pat's symptoms? They include an overwhelming fatigue, headaches, sinus congestion, painful joints, and repeated urinary tract infections. Treated with antibiotics for acne as a teenager, her only current medication is the birth control pill. In order to avoid fats and oils, she relies on soy sauce, vinegar, mustard, and tomato sauce for taste appeal. To conform to the recommended 80 percent carbohydrate intake, she eats whole grains, and she replaces meat with pastas. When she gets hungry, she reaches for crackers, pita bread, and muffins. She is taking good care of herself. Why doesn't she feel better? Why can't her doctors find anything wrong?

This woman could be one of the estimated 60 million Americans (or one in three) experiencing symptoms of candidiasis—chronic yeast infections caused by overgrowth of the yeast *Candida albicans*. Her repeated doses of broad-spectrum antibiotics, long-term use of the birth control pill, and a diet high in carbohydrates have created the ideal biological climate in which the candida can flourish and wreak havoc on her health.

(Speaking of climate, my own experience indicates the importance of external climatic factors in candida development. Although I have practiced throughout the nation, the majority of my candida clients came from the San Francisco Bay area. San Francisco is one of my favorite cities, but its damp, rainy climate seems to contribute to flourishing candida. One of my clients with persistent candida found her problems disappeared when she moved to the drier climate of Southern California.)

Perhaps as many as three quarters of patients with candidiasis are women, for the following reasons:

1. Women suffer regular and frequent hormonal changes and imbalances as a result of the menstrual cycle, the birth control pill, and pregnancy. Such disturbances allow yeasts to grow.

2. The structure of the vagina offers a perfect home for yeasts—dark, moist recesses.

3. The structure of the female bladder and urethra is prone to infection, which is then treated with antibiotics (known activators of yeast growth).

4. Teenage girls are especially concerned about their complexion and may seek antibiotic treatment for acne.

5. Women, in general, are more likely than men to seek treatment from a physician, for everything from throat infections to menstrual difficulties, and are therefore more likely to be treated with antibiotics.

Candida is a Jekyll and Hyde microorganism. How does this friendly, ever-present inhabitant of our gastrointestinal system change into the source of ill health literally from our head to our toes?

Candida is a yeast, part of the huge Fungi kingdom. Molds, mushrooms, mildew, and puffballs are members of the same kingdom.

Even in good health, we carry hundreds of types of yeasts and fungi—over 300 on our skin alone. The most prolific is the yeast *Candida albicans,* which prefers the gastrointestinal tract and genital area.

Normally, all these microbes live in a balanced harmony, producing antibodies that keep other species in check in conjunction with various activities of the immune system.

However, when the circumstances are right candida proliferates. As its numbers grow, the noninvasive yeast changes to a fungus, which bores its rootlike structures into the gastrointestinal mucosa. This allows the fungus, its toxins, and partially digested proteins into the bloodstream—and into every part of the body.

The symptoms that develop depend on the location of the yeast overgrowth and of the concentrations of toxins. Some symptoms include:

- **Gastrointestinal:** indigestion, constipation, diarrhea, abdominal pain, gastritis, bloating, mucus in stool
- **Skin:** itching, scaliness, acne, rashes
- **Eyes:** burning, blurred or erratic vision, chronic inflammation, tearing
- **Ears:** pain, deafness, fluid in ears, recurrent infection
- **Nose and sinuses:** nasal congestion, itching
- **Mouth and throat:** white patches, dry mouth, rash, sore or bleeding gums
- **Urinary/vaginal system:** recurrent bladder infection,

burning or urgent urination, cystitis, vaginal burning, menstrual cramping, irregularities in period, premenstrual anxiety or depression

- **General:** fatigue, loss of body hair, insomnia, weight loss or gain, loss of appetite, irritability, sudden mood swings, agitation, headaches, jittery behavior

Although candidiasis was described by Hippocrates in 400 B.C., it has been the recent work of physicians and researchers such as C. Orian Truss, M.D., a Birmingham, Alabama, physician specializing in diagnosing and treating candidiasis, that has begun to shed light on the factors that permit or encourage yeast overgrowth. These factors include:

A weakened immune system. In 1985 Steven S. Witkin, Ph.D., published in the journal *Infections in Medicine* results of a clinical study of 50 women with recurrent candida vaginal infections. He suggested that the candida infection itself appeared to decrease the body's ability to fight off future infections.[3] In fact, repeated stresses of any kind can eventually weaken the immune system. The immune system may also be deliberately weakened by steroids and other immunosuppressive drugs. Often prescribed for life-threatening or extremely debilitating conditions, such as cancer and arthritis, these drugs nevertheless carry the side effect of allowing yeasts to flourish.

Repeated treatment with broad-spectrum antibiotics. These contribute to yeast overgrowth not only by affecting the immune system by decreasing the ability of white blood cells to destroy germ cells, but also by killing off the friendly, competitive microorganisms along with the disease-causing ones. This imbalance affects the acidity of the intestinal tract and makes additional nutrients available for more yeasts, including the bacteria killed by the drug.

Excess sugar and carbohydrates. First, when simple sugars are consumed, blood sugar (glucose) levels rise quickly and the body produces insulin to carry this glucose to the cells. When blood sugar is too high, the defending cells of the immune system become semiparalyzed. These repeated stresses on our immunity eventually break it down and yeasts begin to overgrow.

Second, sugars, including those found in fruit and starches such as potatoes and rice, are favorite foods of yeasts. Yeast cells grow and multiply rapidly in all sugars. Thus, eating sugary foods increases the likelihood that you are consuming more yeast, as well as providing food for your internal yeast cells. In addition, if carbohydrates are not fully absorbed during digestion, excesses remain in the intestine, once again providing a fertile environment for yeast.

Birth control pills. One common side effect of the use of birth control pills is vaginal yeast infections. High levels of progesterone, present in the Pill, during pregnancy, and during the two-week period prior to menstruation, are believed to change the mucosal membrane of the vagina. These changes encourage the ever-present yeasts to overgrow.

Metabolic factors. Some experts believe that various metabolic factors encourage yeast overgrowth. For example, since copper has fungicidal properties, a deficiency or, more commonly, biounavailability of copper prevents it from acting. Copper is biounavailable when it is present in our systems, but our body cannot process and use it. A stress-induced deficiency of zinc may bring this about, as may a lack of adrenal gland hormones.

Malfunctioning of any of the endocrine glands, including the thyroid as well as the adrenal glands, is thought to be a factor in some cases, besides those related to copper deficiencies. The immune system becomes ineffective after the repeated stress of hormonal imbalance, and once again yeast flourishes.

Biotin, one of the B vitamins, has been shown to prevent the yeast from converting to the harmful fungal form.

Fatty acid deficiency. Japanese researchers have found that oleic acid interferes with the yeast conversion to fungus. This monounsaturated fatty acid is found especially in olive, high-oleic sunflower and safflower, and avocado oils, and to a lesser degree in almond, apricot kernel, canola, peanut, and sesame oils.

In addition, by incorporating into the structure of the cellular membrane, the essential fatty acids decrease the permeability of vital tissues and organs. EFAs prevent yeast from spreading into the bloodstream from its normal intestinal and/or vaginal environs. The yeast cannot pass through the intestinal wall into the circulatory system when the mucous membrane lining of the digestive tract is strengthened by EFAs.

Clinical studies by Dr. Truss have found significant abnormalities in both the Omega 3 and Omega 6 EFAs in patients with candidiasis. He also found evidence of defects in red blood cell outer membranes in the same patients. The red blood cells of his candida patients did not pass through the microscopic pores of a filter as well as did normal red blood cells, indicating rigid outer membranes.

Is Candida Your Problem?

Candidiasis is not a disease that can or should be self-diagnosed. However, because *Candida albicans* is so widespread, standard laboratory tests are not always definitive. The best way for you and your physician to diagnose it may be a combination of reviewing medical history and symptoms with a trial of therapy.

The questionnaire printed below will help you and your physician pinpoint candida's role in your current health; it will not give you a final "yes" or "no" answer. It was prepared for use with adults by William Crook, M.D., a Jackson, Tennessee, allergist, lecturer, and author of several books, including the popular *The Yeast Connection*.

Candida Questionnaire and Score Sheet

For each "yes" answer in Section A, circle the Point Score in that section. Total your score and record it in the box at the end of the section. Then move on to sections B and C and score as directed.

Section A: HISTORY

		Point Score
1.	Have you taken tetracyclines (Sumycin, Panmycin, Vibramycin, Minocin, etc.) or other antibiotics for acne for 1 month (or longer)?	35
2.	Have you, at any time in your life, taken other "broad-spectrum" antibiotics* for respiratory, urinary, or other infections (for 2 months or longer, or in shorter courses 4 or more times in a 1-year period)?	35

3. Have you taken a broad-spectrum antibiotic drug*—even a single course?   6

4. Have you, at any time in your life, been bothered by persistent vaginitis or other problems affecting your reproductive organs?   25

5. Have you been pregnant . . .
2 or more times?   5
1 time?   3

6. Have you taken birth control pills . . .
For more than 2 years?   15
For 6 months to 2 years?   8

7. Have you taken prednisone, Decadron, or other cortisone-type drugs . . .
For more than 2 weeks?   15
For 2 weeks or less?   6

8. Does exposure to perfumes, insecticides, fabric shop odors, and other chemicals provoke . . .
Moderate to severe symptoms?   20
Mild symptoms   5

9. Are your symptoms worse on damp, muggy days or in moldy places?   20

10. Have you had athlete's foot, ringworm, or other chronic fungus infections of the skin or nails? Have such infections been . . .
Severe or persistent?   20
Mild to moderate?   10

11. Do you crave sugar?   10

12. Do you crave breads?   10

13. Do you crave alcoholic beverages?   10

14. Does tobacco smoke *really* bother you?   10

Total score, Section A   _____

---

*Keflex, ampicillin, amoxicillin, Ceclor, Bactrim, or Septra.

Section B: MAJOR SYMPTOMS

For each of your symptoms, enter the appropriate figure in the Point Score column:

If a symptom is occasional or mild, score   3 points

If a symptom is frequent and/or moderately
    severe, score   6 points

If a symptom is severe and/or disabling, score   9 points

Add total score and record it in the box at the end of this
    section.

		Point Score
1.	Fatigue or lethargy	_____
2.	Feeling of being "drained"	_____
3.	Depression	_____
4.	Poor memory	_____
5.	Feeling "spacy" or "unreal"	_____
6.	Inability to make decisions	_____
7.	Numbness, burning, or tingling	_____
8.	Headache	_____
9.	Muscle aches	_____
10.	Muscle weakness or paralysis	_____
11.	Pain and/or swelling in joints	_____
12.	Abdominal pain	_____
13.	Constipation and/or diarrhea	_____
14.	Bloating, belching, or intestinal gas	_____
15.	Troublesome vaginal burning, itching, or discharge	_____
16.	Loss of sexual desire or feeling	_____
17.	Endometriosis or infertility	_____

18. Cramps and/or other menstrual
    irregularities _____
19. Premenstrual tension _____
20. Attacks of anxiety or crying _____
21. Cold hands or feet and/or chilliness _____
22. Shaking or irritable when hungry _____
    Total score, Section B _____

Section C: OTHER SYMPTOMS**

For each of your symptoms, enter the appropriate figure in
the Point Score column:

If a symptom is occasional or mild, score	1 point
If a symptom is frequent and/or moderately severe, score	2 points
If a symptom is severe and/or disabling, score	3 points

Add total score and record it in the box at the end of this
section.

		Point Score
1.	Drowsiness	_____
2.	Irritability or jitteriness	_____
3.	Incoordination	_____
4.	Inability to concentrate	_____
5.	Frequent mood swings	_____
6.	Insomnia	_____
7.	Dizziness/loss of balance	_____
8.	Pressure above ears . . . feeling of head swelling	_____
9.	Tendency to bruise easily	_____
10.	Chronic rashes or itching	_____

11. Numbness, tingling   _____

12. Indigestion or heartburn   _____

13. Food sensitivity or intolerance   _____

14. Mucus in stools   _____

15. Rectal itching   _____

16. Dry mouth or throat   _____

17. Rash or blisters in mouth   _____

18. Bad breath   _____

19. Foot, hair, or body odor not relieved by
     washing   _____

20. Nasal congestion or postnasal drip   _____

21. Nasal itching   _____

22. Sore throat   _____

23. Laryngitis, loss of voice   _____

24. Cough or recurrent bronchitis   _____

25. Pain or tightness in chest   _____

26. Wheezing or shortness of breath   _____

27. Urinary frequency or urgency   _____

28. Burning on urination   _____

29. Spots in front of eyes or erratic vision   _____

30. Burning or tearing of eyes   _____

31. Recurrent infections or fluid in ears   _____

32. Ear pain or deafness   _____

     Total score, Section C   _____

**While the symptoms in this section commonly occur in people
with yeast-connected illness, they are also found in other
individuals.

     Total score, Section A   _____

     Total score, Section B   _____

     Total score, Section C   _____

     GRAND TOTAL SCORE   _____

The Grand Total Score will help you and your physician decide if your health problems are yeast-connected. Yeast-connected health problems are *almost certainly* present in women with scores *over 180*. Yeast-connected health problems are *probably* present in women with scores *over 120*. Yeast-connected health problems are *possibly* present in women with scores *over 60*. With scores of less than 60 in women, yeasts are less apt to cause health problems.

Source: William G. Crook, M.D. This questionnaire is available in quantity from Professional Books, P.O. Box 3246, Jackson, TN 38301.

A *Candida* Prescription

In her book, *Candida: A Twentieth Century Disease*, Shirley S. Lorenzani, Ph.D., points out, "It is possible to reverse Candida overgrowth without the use of anti-yeast drugs. In most cases, however, appropriate use of anti-yeast medication gives the body the boost it needs to gain the upper hand in controlling Candida."[4]

The most commonly prescribed anti-yeast drug is nystatin. This is a relatively safe, natural product made from bacterial fermentation. What few side effects have been reported include headaches and "achiness" for several days after starting therapy. While it is considered the most effective of the medications available, it may nevertheless take as long as two years to bring the yeast under control.

Whether or not you and your doctor choose an anti-yeast drug as treatment, there are a variety of nutritional guidelines to follow that have been helpful to many candida sufferers. You may need to experiment to find the right combination for you. Keep in mind that many of my suggestions that appear later in this book will keep yeasts from gaining control once you have corrected the overgrowth.

1. **Avoid foods containing yeasts, molds, and the products of fermentation,** including:

   Brewer's yeast

   Raised baked goods, such as bread, rolls, pastries, pretzels

   Fermented liquors, including wine, beer, whiskey, brandy, gin, rum, vodka, cider

   Malt-containing products, such as cereals, malted milk, and candies

   Vinegar and vinegar-containing foods, such as pickles, mayonnaise, mustard, catsup, green olives, sauerkraut, horseradish, mincemeat

   Condiments like chutney, soy sauce, spices like cinnamon and black pepper, dried herbs, herb tea

   Pickled and smoked meats

   Mushrooms, truffles

   Cheese, sour cream, buttermilk, cottage cheese, cream cheese

   Dried, candied fruits (wash regular fruits fully)

   Fruit juices, except freshly squeezed; canned tomatoes or tomato juice, unless homemade

   Melons, especially cantaloupe

2. **Avoid vitamin supplements that are yeast-based.**

3. **Avoid chronic medications that stimulate yeast growth:** steroids, birth control pills, and broad-spectrum antibiotics. *Note:* If such medication is essential to your health, it should be continued. Do not discontinue any of these medications without consulting your physician.

4. **Avoid excessive carbohydrates,** especially sugars and gluten-rich grains, which provide a food source for the yeast. Substitute rice, millet, buckwheat, corn, amaranth, or quinoa for the gluten-containing wheat, oats, barley, and rye.

5. **Include garlic daily.** In a study reported in *Mycologia* in 1977, researchers concluded that garlic was markedly inhibitory of all isolates of yeast-like fungi tested.[5] In fact, it is the active component in garlic, allicin, that gives it both its odor and its fungicidal properties. Garlic supplements are available (make sure the allicin has been left in) or you can eat 2 to 4 aspirin-size pieces daily (wrapping it in food helps prevent garlic breath).

6. **Supplement with acidophilus.** *Lactobacillus acidophilus* is one of the friendly intestinal bacteria that compete with candida and help keep the yeast under control. Various acidophilus supplements are available. In addition, although the bacterial levels are much lower than in the supplements, plain, low-fat yogurt also adds lactobacillus to your gastrointestinal system. (Frozen yogurt appears to have little, if any, helpful bacteria left since its processing includes a second pasteurization.)

7. **Consider nutrient supplements.** During periods of active yeast overgrowth, certain vitamins and minerals have been found deficient. According to Leo Galland, M.D., assistant clinical professor at the University of Connecticut Health Center, yeast infections affect the way the body handles magnesium, frequently increasing its excretion. In addition, vitamin B_6 is usually deficient.[6]

Food sources for magnesium include green vegetables, nuts, and seafood. Vitamin B_6 is found in organ meats, fish, soybeans, avocados, peanuts, walnuts, bananas, and other fruits.

Biotin, one of the B vitamins, prevents the yeast from converting to its more destructive fungal form. Food sources are egg yolks, organ meats, legumes, and nuts.

Your individual supplement requirements can be determined in consultation with your physician or nutritionist.

8. **Try taheebo.** Also known as Pau d'Arco, this herbal tea is thought to have an antifungal effect. It has proven helpful to many candida sufferers. It is available loose or in bag form in health food stores.

Once you have the candida under control, the food plan I recommend will help it stay that way. The built-in variety in selection of fiber and grain sources will not only protect against yeast infections, but also help prevent problems with gluten intolerance and mineral loss due to excess fiber, as I explain in the next chapter.

Frankly Female: Vitamin Products for Women

My clients have found several remedies helpful. You may want to check with your own physician or health care professional before using any of the items.

The following supplements are available by calling UNIKEY 1–800–888–4353. For those wanting more nutritional background, copies of my first book, *Beyond Pritikin* are also available at the above number.

Paratox 22—This formula is specifically designed to help control fungus and yeast problems. It is a beneficial aid in eliminating Candida Albicans and also helps to eliminate protozoan infection. It can be taken before meals (2 to 4 capsules, depending upon severity of condition) three times a day.

Superoils—This formula contains a combination of the essential fatty acids so necessary for the cardiovascular, immune, reproductive, and central nervous systems. Superoils is a helpful beauty aid in keeping strong nails, lustrous hair, and smooth skin. Adult women and their men can take 2 capsules twice to three times a day.

Supernutrition Female Formula—This formula is a timed release, multiple vitamin and mineral supplement designed to meet the special needs of women. It contains nutritional support for the ovaries, and special herbs, dong quai and red raspberry, that regulate and balance the female hormonal and blood building systems. Female adults take 2 tablets daily. PMS symptoms are reduced with this supplement.

And, for your man . . .

Supernutrition Male Formula—This formula is a timed release, multiple vitamin and mineral supplement designed to meet the special nutritional needs for men. It contains herbs such as ginseng and damiana that help male stamina and virility as well as special glandulars to balance the entire endocrine system. Adult men take 2 tablets daily.

Aqua Flora—This state of the art homeopathic product aids in controlling yeast allergy. It promotes the friendly bacteria.

Balance—Delicious long-term energy bar for meal replacement. Good for weight loss, levels blood sugar, and used by top athletes.

SEVEN

Carbohydrates: When Enough

Is Too Much—Part II

We have become a society of gluten gluttons.

—Richard A. Kunin, M.D., psychiatrist, author

Perhaps no episode better exemplifies what can happen to nutrition buffs than the 1980s rush to oat bran. In 1987, Robert Kowalski published *The 8-Week Cholesterol Cure*, in which he highlighted the value of oat bran in lowering serum cholesterol. Within a year, sales of at least one oat bran cereal rose 600 percent! New cereals appeared almost overnight. Doughnut chains added high-calorie oat bran muffins to their sugar-laden lineup.

Millions of cholesterol-fearing people eagerly embraced this single food item; they enthusiastically added various oat products, not just the bran, to their diet in the belief that if a little is good, a lot is better. Consuming oats and other grains at every meal and as snacks, however, does not lead to health: it can cause malabsorption of essential vitamins and minerals from too much fiber; it can bring about pain, discomfort, and a lifelong intolerance of the gluten-containing grains wheat, oats, rye, and barley.

Following the publication of *Beyond Pritikin*, I received a telephone call from a Florida newspaper reporter wanting an extensive interview. He had purchased the book, preparatory to the review, and after reading it had implemented my suggestions for individuals with symptoms of gluten intolerance. He had stopped eating his daily whole wheat sandwiches; and his chronic stomach pains, from which he had suffered for almost two years since beginning a high-complex-carbohydrate diet, had disappeared almost overnight. His relief over this simple change in his diet was typical of the response of my clients with similar complaints.

Estimates of the prevalence of gluten intolerance vary and most do not include individuals with minor gluten malabsorption or wheat allergies. The American Celiac Society estimates that 1 in 15,000 Americans suffer from full-scale gluten intolerance, also known as celiac disease, sprue, gluten-induced enteropathy, and ideopathic steatorrhea. In England, home of fresh-baked scones, sandwiches, and pastries at daily teatime, the incidence rises to 1 in 300–400 individuals. On the other hand, in Japan, it is so rare that a celiac society doesn't even exist.

The Staff of Life?

Despite this increased interest in oats, wheat remains the overwhelming favorite in terms of use, representing more than 80 percent of our total grain consumption. As I discussed in Chapter Three, several factors have brought about a 20 percent increase in wheat consumption within a 15-year period: expanded vegetarianism, increased interest in pastas and grain-based ethnic cuisines, and a heightened awareness of the value of fiber.

Most important, however, is the versatility of gluten from wheat and other grains in enhancing processed foods. Gluten is a naturally occurring water-soluble complex protein that gives elasticity and extensibility to grain flours and products made with them. Sophisticated food technologists continue to find new uses for gluten including:

- as an adhesive in breading to coat foods
- as a stabilizer and to add "body" to beverages
- as a glaze over meat patties and other processed meats
- as an expander (gluten quickly absorbs about twice its weight in water)
- as a tableting aid in pharmaceuticals.

Gluten is a component of modified food starch, which is used in almost all processed foods. It is needed to make monosodium glutamate (MSG) and other flavor-enhancers. Wheat flour may be hidden in ice cream, catsup, mayonnaise, and even instant coffee.

In his practice, Richard Kunin, M.D., author of *Mega-Nutrition for Women*, has noted that the majority of patients have some kind of symptom related to minor gluten malabsorption. "A one-sided preference for grains can spell trouble for many people because of a relatively common weak link in the metabolic ability to process these grains," he says.

Unable to handle this gluten overload, many of us develop symptoms of minor gluten malabsorption: fatigue, persistent intestinal gas, bloating within a couple of hours of eating, bowel irregularities, frequent diarrhea, and folic acid deficiency. Others of us develop full-scale gluten intolerance with additional symptoms of irritable bowel, weakness, a tendency to bleed, muscle cramps, bone pain, anemia, headache, and poor appetite.

No matter what the severity, gluten intolerance involves an alteration of the cellular lining of the small intestine. Gluten causes the villi of the lining to flatten. Since these fingerlike structures are responsible for absorption of nutrients, when gluten is present, proteins, fats, carbohydrates, iron, calcium, folic acid, and vitamins D and K are not properly absorbed. Major deficiencies can develop. In women, this may mean menstrual irregularities, infertility, osteoporosis, and anemia, in particular.

Untreated gluten intolerance can lead to intestinal cancer or ulceration, and neurological disorders. In fact, a number of studies are being conducted to examine further the observed associations between gluten intolerance and multiple sclerosis, autism, schizophrenia, rheumatoid arthritis, certain skin conditions, and diabetes.[1]

For example, F. Curtis Dohan, M.D., of Eastern Pennsylvania Psychiatric Institute, Philadelphia, has spent the past 20 years investigating schizophrenia and diet. In one study, twice as many patients who were on a diet free of both cereal and milk in a high-security ward were able to return to the minimum-security ward than those who were on a high-cereal diet. As early as 1966, Dr. Dohan noted that psychoses occurred more often in gluten-intolerant individuals than was predicted by chance. In addition, he has reported that certain substances were found in the urine of both schizophrenics and celiacs.

Research from Berkeley, California, indicates that milk and wheat proteins break down into the same sequence of amino acids during digestion. This may account for the observed frequency of lactose intolerance among the gluten intolerant.

Other studies that have analyzed wheat consumption and schizophrenia incidence statistics report that places where wheat is the staple grain experience higher levels of diagnosed schizophrenia than those in which nongluten grains were staples. For example, a study of 65,000 residents of the highlands of New Guinea, where little or no grain is consumed, found only two chronic schizophrenics; in the coastal area of the same country, wheat is a staple in the diet and schizophrenia occurred about three times as often. In Indonesia, populations of adults who ate grains had a schizophrenia rate of 9.7 per 1,000 people, whereas those whose diet did not include grain had no schizophrenia cases.

In my own practice, one patient, a manic-depressive, was referred to me by her psychiatrist for nutritional counseling. Her diet history revealed excessive amounts of gluten-based grains: bagels every morning, muffins as an evening snack, sandwiches as a lunchtime staple, plus, of course, a wide variety of processed foods which often contained wheat flour. Within three weeks of a diet minus gluten-based products, she reported feeling better, able to cope and her mental outlook was markedly improved. She told me that she felt much less confused and "clearer" for the first time in a long time. She was able to make decisions and stick to them. After keeping a detailed diet history for two months, she was able to see for herself that when she cheated, her mental well-being was negatively affected. Keeping wheat-free was essential to her clarity of mind. This patient eventually developed a food service that specialized in healthy foods.

Overcoming Gluten Intolerance

You may be thinking, "I don't eat *that* much grain." However, when you monitor your food intake with a food diary, you may find more than you thought: cereal for breakfast, a muffin at midmorning, two slices of bread on a lunch-time sandwich, pasta with bread at dinner, and cookies before bed, to be repeated with variations day after day. The more processed foods you eat, the greater your intake of hidden gluten as well. It quickly adds up to much more than your system was designed to handle.

Because of the serious long-term consequences of untreated gluten intolerance, it is essential to consult your physician.

Gluten intolerance can develop at any age. Once it is established, it remains for life, although individuals who develop it in childhood may have a remission during adolescence when they can eat gluten foods without symptoms. However, the damage to the lining of the intestine remains, so the body is still unable to absorb nutrients properly. Therefore, it is important to learn what to avoid and what to include in your diet. For individuals with minor malabsorption, skipping wheat, oats, rye, and barley in products such as baked goods, pastas, and cereals may be enough to allay symptoms. Fiber is contained in a variety of complex carbohydrate sources. Vary your grain choices to avoid overload; grains like rice, millet, corn, and buckwheat are tasty, nutritional nongluten alternatives. Starchy vegetables like squash and sweet potatoes can nutritionally replace grain-based dishes, providing fiber, vitamins, and minerals.

For full-scale gluten intolerance, individuals should avoid a wide variety of foods.

Foods to Avoid[2]

Commercial Beverages and Fruit Juices—ale, beer, gin, whiskey, instant coffee, cocoa, drinking chocolate, malted milk powder, Ovaltine, Postum, tomato juice

Baked Goods—all commercial baked goods, including breads, cakes, cookies, crackers, doughnuts, muffins, pancakes, pastries, waffles, bagels, dinner rolls, crispbread, breadcrumbs, matzoh, pretzels, rusks; baking powder

Candy—all filled chocolates, toffees, fudge, caramel, marzipan, chewing gums

Cereals and grains—all cereals containing wheat, barley, rye, or oats; only cereals guaranteed gluten-free should be consumed (puffed rice, crisped rice, and cornflakes are generally safe); dumplings, macaroni, noodles, spaghetti, canned corn, vermicelli, semolina

Dairy Products—synthetic cream, malted milk, cheese spreads

Desserts and Puddings—all pies, dessert mixes, custard powders, instant desserts, rennet powder or tablets, lemon pie filling, lemon/orange curds, lemon powders, trifle and other desserts with cake ingredients

Fats—commercial salad dressings, mayonnaise

Fish—pickled herring and other pickled fish, frozen breaded fish, fish packaged in sauce, fishpaste

Flours—all flours containing the grains of wheat, barley, rye, and oats

Fruit—baby preparations, glacé fruit

Gravies—gravy thickeners and mixes

Ice Cream—all commercial types plus, of course, cones, wafers, crumb toppings

Meats—all commercial preparations containing fillings, such as sausages, luncheon meats, meat pies, mincemeat, frankfurters, meat pastes; canned meat

Sauces and Condiments—thickened sauces, bottled sauces, pickles, anchovy sauce, catsup, horseradish sauce

Snacks—potato chips, french-fried potatoes

Soups—all canned and dried soups, all thickened soups, all creamed soups

Spices—celery salt, chutney, curry powder, mustard

Spreads—fishpaste, meat spread, cheese spreads, processed peanut butter, sandwich spreads

Vegetables—vegetables in sauces, mayonnaise, or cream; baby foods; vegetable mixes

Note that some products are guaranteed gluten-free by the manufacturer. However, so many processed foods contain MSG and other hidden gluten sources that if you have any doubt at all, you should avoid the food.

[2]*Good Food, Gluten Free,* by Hilda Cherry Hills (New Canaan, CT: Keats Publishing, 1986).

While this list may seem long and may contain some standards in your diet, especially if you are a grabber like Maryann or a nutrition buff like Pat, the list of available foods is equally varied. In fact, my Food-Wise Woman Food Plan, with modification of the choice of grains, provides the basis for a healthful, gluten-free life-style.

Foods to Enjoy

Fruits—all fresh or frozen ones; juices except tomato; apple and other fruit sauces; dried. fruits

Vegetables—all fresh, frozen, or canned, as long as they do not have sauces; raw or cooked, including steamed, boiled, roasted

Carbohydrates—whole brown or converted rice, millet, buckwheat, corn, amaranth, quinoa; lentils, dried peas, butter beans; potatoes, parsnips, pumpkin

Proteins—meats, including lean beef, lamb, veal (except as noted above); fish; poultry; cheese; eggs; soya beans

Fats—100 percent expeller-pressed, natural oils

See the shopping list in Chapter Ten for more detailed information on the food staples.

A Note About Nongluten Grains

While gluten-free white flour is available, it is a refined product, devoid of the vitamins, minerals, and fiber of whole grains. Therefore, it is not a recommended substitute. I recommend more emphasis on the gluten-free grains: rice, millet, corn, buckwheat, and the latest on natural food shelves, amaranth, quinoa, teff, and spelt. Ener-G-Foods (distributed through natural food stores nationwide) and Berkshire Mountain Bakery (available on the East Coast) bake gluten-free breads and make varieties that are yeast-free and wheat-free as well. Flours from potatoes, soy, rice, and tapioca can successfully be used in cooking. Gluten-intolerant individuals may find they are intolerant to some or all of these as well, so experiment with your own diet.

Quinoa, known as the Mother Grain of the Incan civilization, contains one of the highest levels of protein of any grain, with an average of 16 percent compared with 14 percent in wheat, 9 percent in millet, and 7 percent in rice. The seed is rich in the amino acid lysine, so helpful in curbing herpes viruses and ridding the body of metabolized lipoproteins. It has the same amount of calcium as lowfat milk, with four times the phosphorus. It is also a good source of B vitamins and vitamin C.

This chart compares quinoa with several gluten and non-gluten grains for its nutritional and dietary fiber content, expressed in percentages.

Nutritional and Fiber Content of Selected Grains

	Water	Protein	Fat	Carbo-hydrates	Fiber	Ash
Quinoa	11.4	16.2	6.9	63.9	3.5	3.3
Wheat	13.0	14.0	2.2	69.1	2.3	1.7
Oats	12.5	13.0	5.4	66.1	10.6	3.0
Rice	12.0	7.5	1.9	77.4	0.9	1.2
Buckwheat	11.0	11.7	2.4	72.9	9.9	2.0

Source: Lupine and Quinoa, by I. Junge (Chile: University of Concepcion Publication, 1973) and U.S.D.A.

After cooking, quinoa quadruples in size, yet retains its crunchiness. It can be used in salads, as a substitute for couscous, as a side dish mixed with pesto, or a stuffing for poultry or vegetables.

It is available from health food and specialty stores; it is imported by: Quinoa Corp., 24248 Crenshaw Blvd., Suite 220, Torrance, CA 90505.

Amaranth is also a South-Central American grain high in protein, measuring some 16–18 percent. It is high in vitamins A, B, and C, calcium, and fiber. Amaranth flour is used in cookies, crusts, crackers, cakes, muffins, pancakes, breads, and pocketbreads. Breakfast cereals are also available that feature amaranth. If your local stores don't carry it, write: Illinois Amaranth Company, Box 464-D, Mundelein, IL 60060.

What About Fiber?

Individuals who currently rely on bran cereals for their fiber may not realize that there are many delicious, inexpensive, gluten-free fiber alternatives. And, yes, there are even alternatives to oat bran that have the same cholesterol-reducing properties.

Fiber is the indigestible part of plant foods. There are several kinds, including pectins, gums, cellulose, and mucilages. Some are insoluble because they do not dissolve in water. Insoluble fibers include the fiber contained in wheat and corn bran, grains, nuts, and some vegetables. Insoluble fibers absorb water as they move through the intestines, increasing the size of the stool. This helps waste materials to move out at a faster pace, a process believed to contribute to the lower rates of colon and rectal cancer among those eating high-fiber diets. The fiber is thought to reduce the time cancer-causing substances spend in the intestines and to dilute their concentration. Insoluble fiber is also helpful in bowel disorders such as constipation and diverticular disease, in which weakened areas of the intestine wall become inflamed.

However, due to its coarseness, too much insoluble fiber may irritate the bowel. Another problem with grain fiber, especially wheat bran, is that it can interfere with the absorption of crucial female minerals, including calcium, magnesium, iron, and zinc. Given the low intake of these minerals by many women, increased secretion stimulated by too much fiber can only add to the likelihood of deficiency and ill-health.

Soluble fiber, which dissolves in water, is rich in pectins and gums. Oat bran, barley, black-eyed peas, fresh vegetables like carrots and okra, fresh fruits like apples, prunes, and grapefruit, are rich sources of soluble fiber.

What about oat bran's cholesterol-reducing powers? It is the soluble fiber in the oats that has been shown to lower cholesterol, in one study by 36 milligrams, in another by 10.6 percent. However, pectin (fruit fiber), psyllium seed husks, and guar gum (a bean fiber) have all proven helpful in lowering blood cholesterol levels in clinical studies.

Other studies have found particular health benefits of soluble fiber for diabetics. For example, James W. Anderson, M.D., of the Veterans Administration Hospital, Lexington, Kentucky, studied the effects of a high-carbohydrate, high-fiber diet on diabetics. He found that when carbohydrates are eaten *with* fiber, the blood sugar levels did not rise as high as when carbohydrates were eaten alone, so the diabetics required less insulin. The fiber slowed the absorption of the carbohydrates.

Another study at the University of Bristol, England, found that fiber lowered the demand for insulin in healthy subjects and produced a longer-lasting feeling of fullness—news for women trying to avoid overeating. When individuals were given apple juice, the insulin level in their blood rose twice as high as that of individuals who ate an equivalent amount of whole apples. Furthermore, by the time blood sugar levels had returned to normal in the whole-apple group, the levels were clearly below normal in the juice group, a response usually associated with hunger pangs.

Fiber Alternatives

The average American diet contains about 10 grams of fiber. Recommended levels are 25 to 35 grams to optimize the cancer-prevention, cholesterol-lowering, and intestinal cleansing effects. A diet that emphasizes un-refined, unprocessed fresh foods, such as the plan de-scribed in this book, will enable you to meet these recommendations without counting grams. Here is a list of the fiber content of various high-fiber, nongluten foods, along with some suggestions for food choices that will increase your intake of dietary fiber.

High-Fiber Foods

Food	Serving Size	Grams Dietary Fiber
Acorn squash, cooked	½ cup	3.6
Almonds, chopped	2 tablespoons	2.2
Apple, with peel	1 medium	2.8
Asparagus, cooked	¾ cup	3.1
Blackberries, fresh	½ cup	4.5
Black-eyed peas, cooked	½ cup	12.4
Broccoli, raw	½ cup	2.5
Brussels sprouts, cooked	½ cup	3.9
Carrots, cooked	½ cup	2.3
Carrots, raw	1 medium	3.7
Corn, vacuum packed	½ cup	6.0
Green beans, cooked	½ cup	2.3
Green peas, young, canned	½ cup	7.9
Kale, cooked	½ cup	2.8
Kidney beans, canned	½ cup	7.9
Lentils, cooked	½ cup	2.0
Nectarine	1 small	1.7
Onion, raw, chopped	½ cup	2.6
Pear, fresh	1 medium	5.0

Food	Serving Size	Grams Dietary Fiber
Pinto beans, cooked	½ cup	5.3
Potato, white, baked with skin	1 medium	3.8
Prunes, cooked	⅓ cup	5.8
Raspberries, red, fresh	¾ cup	6.8
Sauerkraut, canned	½ cup	2.4
Spinach, canned	½ cup	2.5
Spinach, raw	2 large leaves	1.8
Split peas, cooked	½ cup	5.1
Strawberries, fresh	¾ cup	2.0
Sweet potato, cooked	1 large	4.2
Zucchini, cooked, sliced	½ cup	2.7

Source: Adapted from *Plant Fiber in Foods,* by James W. Anderson, M.D. (Lexington, KY: HCF Diabetes Research Foundation).

Fiber Fixes Without the Gluten

- Eat the whole fruit rather than the juice—all the vitamins plus the fiber, with less concentrated sugar.

- High-fiber lunches include lentil, split pea, or black bean soup; vegetarian chili; a bean burrito; or a steamed vegetable plate.

- At the salad bar, look for sprouts, peas, garbanzo beans, raw cauliflower, broccoli, and zucchini to add to your greens.

- A sweet potato has 4.2 grams fiber per potato. Use as a side dish instead of pasta. Try making sweet potato muffins or bread with nongluten flour, instead of oat bran muffins.

- Snack on raw vegetables or air-popped popcorn for a high-fiber fill-up.

- Add pureed vegetables such as beans or peas to thicken sauces or soups.

- Serve fruits and vegetables unpeeled whenever possible. Nutrients as well as fiber are often stored there.

Fiber Choices	
Instead of	*Choose*
white rice	brown rice
apple juice	whole raw apple
hamburger on bun	chili with beans
salami on hard roll	bean taco with lettuce/tomato
chicken noodle soup	lentil soup
lettuce salad	spinach salad
strawberry ice cream	strawberries
macaroni salad	three-bean salad

Fiber has "come out of the closet" and, given the research findings about its health benefits, it deserves to stay out. However, to make the most of these benefits, think of fiber as an integral part of your food choices from unrefined foods and grains, rather than as a separate food additive to be tolerated by sprinkling it on other foods. Gradually replace low-fiber foods with high-fiber ones and you will establish a new eating pattern that you can maintain throughout your life without wreaking havoc on your digestive system.

EIGHT

What Women Miss
About Calcium

*The only way to keep your health is to eat
what you don't want, drink what you don't like and do
what you'd rather not.*

—Mark Twain

An estimated three quarters of American women over age 35 do not get the recommended 1,000 milligrams of calcium every day. They risk gum disease, menstrual cramping, depression, insomnia, and, in their futures, osteoporosis, the brittle bone disease. If we briefly review the three diet styles I have referred to throughout this book, I think you'll see why such a deficiency exists.

Susan, the chronic dieter, takes in fewer calories and, of course, fewer nutrients than her nondieting colleagues. She skips the calories of dairy products for the zero calories of diet soft drinks. Should her dieting begin to affect her menstrual cycle, she could experience disruptions in estrogen production. Low dietary intake of calcium, magnesium, and boron; low estrogen levels; and excess phosphorus, from the soft drinks, are all negative factors in the complex process of calcium absorption.

The nutrition buff, Pat, has her share of calcium disrupters. Embracing the high-carbohydrate, low-fat dietary model of the 1980s, she, too, avoids dairy products. While she gets some alternative calcium sources in her vegetables, the oxalic acid in several of them and the phytic acid in the many grains she eats work to inhibit calcium absorption.

Grabbers like Maryann tend to eat too much salt, caffeine, "bad" fats, and sugar. The processed foods they reach for are frequently deficient in the calcium-aiding nutrients magnesium, boron, and vitamins C, D, and K. As I will explain, all of these factors, along with several others, affect the body's ability to use 'what calcium is present, contributing to postmenopausal osteoporosis.

Putting Calcium to Use: How It Works

No matter how much calcium you take in, a certain amount will pass through the intestine and kidneys and be lost through excretion. This process protects the neuromuscular system, preventing muscle spasm. In addition, the level of calcium carried in the blood at all times must stay between 9 and 11 milligrams per 100 cubic centimeters of blood. This means that if calcium intake is low, the body must get calcium from another source in order to maintain the blood calcium level.

When blood calcium levels drop, the parathyroid gland sends out a hormone which signals "bone breakers" to release calcium being stored in the bones. This calcium restores the level in the blood to normal.

If calcium levels are too high, another hormone stimulates production of bone cells, which ties up the excess calcium.

While 99 percent of our body's calcium is in our bones, the other one percent circulating in our blood, fluids, and within our soft tissue is critical to the proper functioning of every cell. This accounts for the complex system designed to maintain these calcium levels, no matter what our dietary intake. Calcium plays a critical role in blood clotting, cell division, muscle contractions and maintenance of tone, brain function, hormonal balance, and even our heartbeat. It has a sedative effect (remember mom's glass of warm milk before bed!) and serves as a nerve tranquilizer. Research at the New York Hospital–Cornell Medical Center has found that calcium can lower blood pressure in certain individuals. Other studies point to a lower risk of colon cancer with adequate calcium levels.

The body cannot manufacture calcium, so the mineral must come from our diet or supplements. Symptoms of severe blood calcium deficiency include painful muscle contractions, tremors, and convulsions; lesser deficiencies may bring on heart palpitations, backaches, bone pain, insomnia, numbness, and menstrual cramps. Inflamed and bleeding gums (other than those caused by a vitamin C deficiency) are frequently an early warning sign of significant depletion of bone calcium—osteoporosis.

The Inhibitors

Even if you take in the recommended amounts of calcium in your diet, certain factors can affect calcium metabolism and absorption, causing calcium deficiency. These factors include:

- Diet that is high in fat, protein, or sodium
- Imbalances in the calcium-phosphorus ratio
- Aluminum intake
- Oxalates from cocoa, dandelion greens, sorrel, rhubarb, and spinach
- Phytic acid and excess fiber from grains and bran
- Caffeine
- Cigarette smoking
- Inadequate hydrochloric acid in the stomach for digestion
- Certain drugs and over-the-counter medications

Excesses in Diet

A high-protein diet brings excess nitrogen and sulfur into the blood, which sets up an acid condition that leaches calcium from the bone to neutralize the condition. High levels of the wrong fats combine with calcium in the intestines, forming insoluble compounds that make the calcium unusable. Excess sodium causes calcium to be excreted in urine; this, in turn, lowers blood calcium levels, signaling the hormone system to cause calcium to be withdrawn from bones.

Calcium-Phosphorus Balance

The calcium-phosphorus ratio is a vital factor in the optimal use of calcium. About one fourth of the mineral content of your body is phosphorus, most of it tied up as calcium phosphate. Experts believe we need approximately a 1.2:1 ratio of calcium to phosphorus (an average of 1,000 milligrams calcium to 800 milligrams phosphorus daily) to keep the calcium absorption process in balance. Too much sugar lowers the blood phosphorus level. Excesses in phosphorus build up in a diet high in red meat, poultry, and carbonated soft drink consumption. Meats like pork chops and ham contain up to 30 times more phosphorus than calcium. Chicken contains more phosphorus (250 milligrams in 3½ ounces) than even lean cuts of red meat (158 milligrams in 3½ ounces of ground lean beef).

Soft drinks contain phosphoric acid, a phosphorus-containing substance that puts bubbles in the beverages. The soda does not, however, contain an equivalent amount of calcium to maintain the necessary calcium-phosphorus balance. Soft drinks containing the highest levels of phosphates include Tab, Diet Coke, Coca-Cola, Caffeine-Free Coke, and Mr. Bibb.

Aluminum

Aluminum affects both phosphorus and calcium. According to a 1975 article in *Gastroenterology*, small amounts of aluminum-containing antacids, taken 3–4 times a day for 2–5 weeks, inhibited absorption of phosphorus and increased the excretion of calcium in urine and feces, especially in individuals with low calcium intake.[1] Taking more than two teaspoons of these antacids a day can begin to affect your calcium levels.

It is interesting to note that some antacids like TUMS are, however, good sources of calcium. TUMS contains calcium carbonate, but no aluminum. Its use as a supplement should be moderated, though, since it contains both sucrose and talc.

Aluminum is found in many antacids (Maalox, Amphojel, Gelusil, Mylanta); in foods cooked in aluminum pans or wrapped in foil; in beverages served in aluminum cans; in many local drinking water supplies (fluoridation adds to the problem by leaching aluminum into the water from the surrounding storage areas); in pickles; in peppermint tea; and in processed cheeses, cheese spreads, and cream cheese.

Oxalates and Phytates

Some foods contain natural substances that interfere with calcium absorption. For example, spinach is high in calcium, but it contains calcium-blocking oxalates. So do cocoa, asparagus, sorrel, rhubarb, and dandelion greens. The oxalic acid they contain binds with the calcium to form calcium oxalate, which is indigestible.

Grains have phytic acid, a phosphorus-like compound which combines with calcium in the intestine and blocks its absorption. In excess (as in some vegetarian and high-carbohydrate diets), grains also provide too much insoluble fiber, which binds with the calcium and carries it out of the body, unused. Try to avoid high-oxalate and phytic acid foods with calcium-rich meals.

Caffeine

Caffeine, from coffee, tea, and soft drinks, doubles the rate of calcium excretion. Three cups of black coffee can result in a 45-milligram calcium loss.

Cigarette Smoking

In her book, *The Calcium Plus Workbook*, Evelyn Whitlock, M.D., highlights the role of cigarette smoking: "Smoking doubles the risk of osteoporosis, decreases the effectiveness of estrogen, is associated with early menopause and worsens the detrimental effects of chronic underweight on the skeleton. The bad news about smoking just keeps getting worse!"[2]

In several recent studies three quarters of the women who developed osteoporosis are or were smokers, most of whom smoked at least a pack a day. Some animal studies have shown demineralization of bone when there are high blood levels of cadmium, such as that found in the blood of cigarette smokers. Other studies point to the altered level of estrogen and other hormones brought about by cigarettes. Women who smoke a pack a day begin menopause an average of 2 years earlier than non-smokers.

Hydrochloric Acid

As we age, our ability to absorb calcium declines: in women, this process begins in their 40s, in men not until their 60s. Our bodies also produce less hydrochloric acid. A study by Drs. Robert Heaney and Robert Recker of Creighton University, Omaha, found poor calcium absorption in middle-aged women who did not secrete adequate stomach acid.

Consumption of carbonated soft drinks can contribute to this problem in women of all ages. The beverages neutralize hydrochloric acid, thereby making it ineffective for digestion and calcium absorption.

Drugs and Calcium

A number of drugs have been found to interact with calcium or its enhancer, vitamin D. Some act to increase excretion, others block absorption. Here are the common ones:

Calcium and Vitamin D Effects of Common Prescription Drugs

Drug	Calcium Effect	Vit. D Effect
Anticonvulsants		
Dilantin	*	Decreased absorption

Drug	Calcium Effect	Vit. D Effect
Phenobarbital	*	Increased inactivation
Primidone	*	Increased inactivation
Sedatives		
Glutethimide	*	Decreased absorption, increased in-activation
Antacids		
Aluminum hydroxide	Increased urinary excretion	Can cause vitamin D deficiency
Maalox or Mylanta	Decreased absorption	—
Laxatives		
Mineral oil	*	Decreased absorption
Phenolphthalein	Decreased absorption	Decreased absorption
Steroids		
	Decreased absorption, increased excretion, decreased bone formation, increased bone breakdown	Decreased activation
Diuretics		
Furosemide, Ethacrynic acid, Triamterene	Increased urinary excretion	—

Drug	Calcium Effect	Vit. D Effect
Thiazide (chloro- or hydrochloro-)	Lowered urinary calcium	—
Thyroid hormone	Increased urinary excretion, increased loss in sweat	—
Tetracycline	Decreased absorption	—
Vitamin A (75,000 IU)	Increased urinary loss	—
Cholestyramine	*	Decreased absorption
Para-amino salicylic acid	?	May cause vitamin D malabsorption from fat malabsorption
Methotrexate	Calcium loss	—
Sulfur-containing amino acids	Increased urinary loss	—

Source: *The Calcium Plus Workbook,* by Evelyn P. Whitlock, M.D. (New Canaan, CT: Keats Publishing, 1988). Copyright 1988 by Evelyn P. Whitlock.

*May show decreased absorption due to vitamin D effects.

The Enhancers

With so many inhibitors, it is not surprising that as many as 24 million Americans suffer from osteoporosis brought on by inadequate calcium. However, there are several enhancers of calcium absorption, including:

- vitamins C, D, and K
- magnesium
- trace minerals boron and silicon
- estrogen
- exercise

The Enhancing Vitamins

Several vitamins are valuable for adequate calcium absorption. Vitamin C is one enhancer. Vitamin D is essential for calcium to be transformed into a usable form. It increases calcium absorption in the small intestine and calcium retention by the kidneys, and it helps the action of the parathyroid hormone to release calcium from the bone. Vitamin D is made in the skin, with the help of the essential fatty acids, in the presence of sunlight. Spending one hour in the sun will produce about 600 units of vitamin D, more than the recommended daily allowance. (There are a number of drugs that interfere with vitamin D; see the chart on pages 116–118.)

Preliminary studies indicate a role for vitamin K in maintaining bone strength. A report in *The Journal of Clinical Endocrinology and Metabolism* indicates that people with osteoporosis had low levels of vitamin K. When levels were normalized, bone density increased and bone loss decreased.[3]

Magnesium

Magnesium acts in concert with calcium and phosphorus. It is vital for calcium metabolism and transport into bone and soft tissues; it helps prevent formation of calcium oxalate crystals (kidney stones). Some researchers have suggested a ratio of one part magnesium to two parts calcium for optimal bone health.

The Enhancing Trace Elements

As research into osteoporosis and bone fragility continues, new relationships begin to emerge, albeit not always clearly defined. For example, a recent study by the U.S. Department of Agriculture found that after eight days of 3-milligram supplements of boron, the postmenopausal women studied lost 40 percent less calcium, 33 percent less magnesium, and slightly less phosphorus.[4] Finding double the prestudy blood levels of the most active form of estrogen, researchers suggest that boron is necessary for the synthesis of estrogen, vitamin D, and other steroid hormones. More research may pinpoint further the role of this trace element.

Another trace element, silicon, is also known to influence calcium uptake in bones.

Estrogen

Estrogen, one of the sex hormones, is integral to the body's efficient use of calcium. Estrogen both increases calcium absorption and decreases its urinary excretion. Any activity or illness that lowers estrogen levels, triggering loss of menstruation, can bring on significant bone loss, especially from the spine. Very low calorie diets (500 calories), excessive exercise, and anorexia (an eating disorder) are some of these activities. When these activities cause women who are very thin to stop having a menstrual cycle for a year or more, the most bone loss occurs.

The Special Role of Exercise

The goal for premenopausal women is to build the strongest bone possible during their 20s and early 30s and then maintain this bone from about age 35, when bone building stops, to menopause, when estrogen production declines. Some bone loss is inevitable with age— as early as age 25, women begin losing bone at the rate of one percent per year—but it does not have to lead to injury and even death from osteoporosis.

Knowing that calcium won't cure osteoporosis or even prevent bone loss when considered alone, researchers are looking for combinations of factors that can at least slow, if not stop, bone loss. Weight-bearing exercise appears to be one element of the formula.

Bones become stronger with physical stress. If they are not used, they lose calcium and become porous. In addition, by strengthening the muscles and tendons that protectively surround bone, exercise makes bones less susceptible to injury.

A recent study from the Mayo Clinic found that as much as one half of all spongy bone, like that of the spine, is lost *before* menopause. Weight-bearing exercise is especially effective in building this type of bone in women under age 35.

There's more:

- "Women who exercise twice a week have denser bones than those who exercise once a week, who in turn have denser bones than those who never exercise at all," writes Dr. Whitlock in *The Calcium Plus Workbook*.[5]

- Even sedentary postmenopausal women increased bone mass by five percent after a nine-month exercise program and high-calcium diet.

- Another study found that individuals who walked aerobically retained much more bone mass than those who rode a stationary bicycle or worked out on Nautilus.

Weight-bearing exercises are those that cause your muscles to pull on bones to move some or all of your body or objects you carry through space or against gravity. That means walking, jogging, running, tennis, skiing, hiking, jumping rope, and aerobic dancing. The bone-building effects of lifting weights and trampolining are still being studied. The form of exercise you choose depends on your interests, your physical condition, the cost, and convenience. (It's wise to consult your physician before beginning any exercise program.)

Although research continues to find the optimal exercise program for bone fitness, Dr. Whitlock makes the following suggestions:

1. Exercise at least 3 times a week for 20–60 minutes at a low to medium intensity.

2. Activity should be weight-bearing, as described above.

3. Activity should involve pulls on a variety of muscles.

4. Choose activities you enjoy so you are more likely to continue.

5. Include warm-up and cool-down exercises for about five minutes each—slow stretches and bends that will prepare your muscles for the change of pace.

6. Choose a program that is nontraumatic to your bones and muscles. Consider your physical condition and the shape your bones are in—you don't have to walk four miles the first day.

7. Make sure you have good equipment—well-made walking shoes, for instance. These will help avoid injury and discomfort.

Remember, if you are a premenopausal woman, don't exercise so much that you cause your periods to stop—this causes more harm than good.

The Risk of Osteoporosis

Osteoporosis affects half the women over age 45. The brittle weakening of the bones results, for example, in twice as many women as men suffering hip fractures. The risk factors for developing the disease include:

- **Heredity**—women with female relatives who have osteoporosis are more likely to develop it.
- **Sex**—women's bones are less dense than men's; women tend to take in 50 percent less calcium than men due to food selection and frequent dieting; women live longer than men, so there is more time for the bone loss to take effect (a double-edged sword!).
- **Onset of menopause**—the earlier the onset, the greater the risk of osteoporosis.
- **Ethnic background**—women with ancestors from the British Isles, northern Europe, China, or Japan have the highest risk.
- **Stature and build**—short or medium-height women have the greater risk; slender or excessively thin women have less dense bones than obese women, so feel the bone loss more.
- **Certain diseases**—endocrine disorders, diabetes, and rheumatoid arthritis put women at risk.

- **Cigarette smoking.**
- **Inadequate calcium levels** (as described earlier in this chapter).
- **Inadequate exercise** (see above).

A Diet for Fit Bones

The current recommended daily allowances (in milligrams, unless noted) for women of the several "bone builders" are:

	Calcium	Phosphorus	Magnesium	Boron*
over age 25	800	800	280	1–2
pregnant	1,200	1,200	300	1–2
lactating	1,200	1,200	355	1–2

	Vitamin C	Vitamin D**	Vitamin K**
over age 25	60	5	65
pregnant	70	10	65
lactating	95	10	65

Source: Based on data in *Recommended Dietary Allowances*, 10th edition (Washington, D.C.: National Academy of Sciences, 1989) and other sources.

*Estimates. Values for silicon undetermined.

**Micrograms.

These nutrients are found in a variety of foods as suggested below.

Sources of Bone-Builder Nutrients

Calcium

Item	Serving size	Calcium (milligrams)
yogurt, plain low-fat	1 cup	415
sardines, with bones	3 ounces	372
ricotta, part skim	½ cup	337
skim milk	1 cup	302
buttermilk	1 cup	300
whole sesame seeds	3 table- spoons	300
whole milk	1 cup	291
Swiss cheese	1 ounce	262
turnip greens, cooked	1 cup	250
bok choy, cooked	1 cup	250
cheddar cheese	1 ounce	213
oysters, raw	¾ cup	170
salmon, canned with bones	3 ounces	167
beans, garbanzo, cooked	1 cup	150
molasses, blackstrap	1 table- spoon	150
almonds	½ cup	150
mustard greens, cooked	½ cup	97
corn muffin	2 medium	90
cottage cheese, 2 percent fat	½ cup	77
kale, cooked	½ cup	74
broccoli, cooked	½ cup	68
orange	1 medium	54
mineral waters (1 liter servings):		
Contrexeville		451

Item	Serving size	Calcium (milligrams)
Mendocino		380
San Pellegrino		200
Perrier		140
Apollinaris		91

Source: Based on data from *Agriculture Handbook* Nos. 8 and 456 (Washington, DC: US Government Printing Office) and other sources.

Phosphorus
meat, poultry, eggs, fish, dried peas and beans, dairy products, whole grains, carbonated soft drinks

Magnesium
raw leafy greens, nuts, seeds, whole grains, soybeans

Boron
fruits and vegetables, especially apples and pears; green leafy vegetables; legumes; nuts

Silicon
alfalfa, oat bran, wheat bran, soybean meal

Vitamin C
citrus fruits, melon, strawberries, tomatoes, green peppers, broccoli, brussels sprouts, potatoes, dark green vegetables

Vitamin D
fish oils, beef, butter, eggs, fortified nonfat milk, salmon, tuna

Vitamin K
leafy greens, peas, potatoes, cabbage, liver, cereals

The sample one-week menu plan outlined in Chapter Twelve has been designed to enhance your calcium intake. I've also included a number of hints on ways to increase your dietary calcium effortlessly.

Supplementing Calcium

Your choices determine how "calcium healthy" you are—you *can* get adequate levels of calcium and its enhancers from your diet by choosing to include some dairy products and a variety of other foods.

However, for postmenopausal women, whose calcium needs many experts believe rise to 1,500 milligrams daily; for pregnant and lactating women; and for any woman who doubts her ability to get a full level of calcium on most days, supplements can be a reassurance.

Supplements should do just that—supplement dietary sources, not replace them. If you have already reviewed your diet (perhaps the food diary described in Chapter Two will help) and estimate that you are getting about 600 milligrams of calcium, then a 200-milligram supplement, not the full 800-milligram daily allowance, will be adequate and safe.

I have described the complex interactions between calcium, its inhibitors, and its enhancers. The bioavailability of the calcium is the key—you are only throwing money away if you take calcium supplements and continue to drink coffee or soft drinks, smoke cigarettes, or avoid exercise. Remove the inhibitors, introduce or increase the enhancers, and then and only then consider your supplemental needs (see also Chapter Eight).

Calcium is unstable alone, so supplements must be made with calcium in combination with other minerals. The most common are:

- calcium carbonate—from oyster shells, with 40 percent calcium
- calcium citrate—24 percent calcium
- calcium lactate—from milk sugar, which should be avoided by lactose intolerant individuals, 13 percent calcium
- calcium gluconate—9 percent calcium
- calcium glubionate—6.5 percent calcium

Calcium phosphate contains over 23 percent calcium, but is not generally recommended, since our diets tend to have excessive phosphorus. Bone meal (31 percent calcium) and dolomite (22 percent calcium) should also be avoided since they may be contaminated with lead and other toxic minerals.

A number of studies have been performed to try to determine which form is most effective. In 1987, Ralph Shangraw, chairman of the Department of Pharmaceutics at the University of Maryland School of Pharmacy, published the results of his analysis of 80 calcium supplements. He found that almost half of the various brands did not disintegrate and the calcium went unused.[6]

Earlier, researchers from the University of Texas Health Sciences Center at Dallas concluded that "calcium citrate provides a more optimum calcium bioavailability than calcium carbonate." The same year, 1985,

Robert Recker, M.D., of Creighton University, Omaha, reported in *The New England Journal of Medicine* that the calcium in citrate form was significantly better absorbed by individuals with low levels of stomach acid (common in women over 40) than was the calcium in the carbonate form.[7]

Use the recommended daily allowance chart in the previous section as a guide to your need for supplementation of any or all of the "bone builders." Remember, this is *not* a case for "a little is good, a lot is better." Balance, from varied natural food sources wherever possible, is the key to a lifetime of strong bones.

NINE

Are There

"Female" Minerals?

*The physician has but a single task: to cure; and if he
succeeds, it matters not a whit by what means he has succeeded.*

—Hippocrates

All of us, men and women alike, are made up of organic
elements—primarily oxygen, carbon, hydrogen, and nitrogen—and inorganic minerals such as calcium and potassium. These minerals supply no calories, but they are
essential. Michael Lesser, M.D., in *Nutrition and Vitamin
Therapy*, emphasizes, "Humans can tolerate a deficiency
of vitamins longer than a deficiency of minerals. A slight
change in the blood's level of important minerals may
rapidly endanger health and survival."[1]

While it is true, then, that both sexes can feel the
effects of mineral deficiencies, it is also true that women
are more likely to be deficient. The chronic dieter, the
nutrition buff, and the grabber are each in her own way
at risk of deficiency.

Richard Kunin, M.D., San Francisco–based author
of *Mega-Nutrition for Women*, writes, "The differences

between a man's and a woman's biochemistry are so profound that it is a national scandal that we act as if a woman can be healthy on a male diet. . . . From month to month, from birth to the giving of life to the change of life, women face a unique challenge to keep their body chemistry in balance."[2]

I believe the answer to the question, "Are there 'female' minerals?" has to be, "Yes." They are: calcium, phosphorus, and magnesium, known as bulk or macrominerals because they are present in relatively large quantities in our bodies; and the trace or microminerals (each comprising less than 0.01 percent of our total body weight) iron, zinc, manganese, iodine, and copper. Some of these we have already discussed in detail.

Besides calcium and phosphorus, there is another mineral critical for health. Magnesium is responsible for more biochemical reactions in the body than any other mineral. It tunes up all cells, tissues, and organs—getting the body ready for productive activity and wear and tear. It is the mineral cofactor in DNA cell rebuilding and plays an important role in neuromuscular problems, the cardiac muscle, smooth muscle tissue, nerve impulse transmission, and the metabolism of carbohydrates and amino acids. Magnesium acts as a natural tranquilizer and reduces tremors and cramps. It is a major mineral cofactor in the tranformation of essential fats into prostaglandins, those extraordinarily powerful compounds that control all bodily function on a cellular level.

Magnesium has been found by researchers at the University of California to be low in the blood of many women prior to and during their period. Some women have found it helpful in relieving the symptoms of premenstrual syndrome (see below for more on PMS).

Magnesium appears to be especially important to

pregnant women. A study published in the *British Journal of Obstetrics and Gynecology* in 1988 reports that, compared to a nonsupplemented control group, women given 360 milligrams of supplemental magnesium daily from the third month of pregnancy:[3]

- were less likely to hemorrhage;
- had fewer cervical problems;
- retained less fluid; and
- were more likely to deliver normal-size, responsive babies.

Other researchers have found that magnesium levels are low in depressed individuals and rise after recovery. The magnesium in the cells, not in the blood, decreases and may account for the symptoms. Furthermore, low levels of both blood and cellular magnesium have been reported in individuals with high blood pressure.

Women who take the birth control pill should be especially watchful of their magnesium intake, since this medication decreases the mineral in the bloodstream.

Magnesium is the third partner in the bone-building process and is subject to the effects of inhibitors just as calcium and phosphorus are. Preferably, the diet should provide two parts calcium for each one part of magnesium. Alcohol; high levels of protein, fat, calcium, phosphorus, or phytic acid; and synthetic vitamin D (as in fortified milk) can negatively affect the mineral's availability within the body.

The RDA for women is:

19 and over	280 milligrams
pregnant or lactating	300 or 355 milligrams

Food sources include: raw leafy greens, sea vegetables, almonds, sunflower seeds, whole grains, blackstrap molasses, and soybeans.

Trace Minerals for Women

Iron

While our bodies contain only about 4 grams of iron, over half of which is in the red blood cells, it is vital to every tissue in the body. As a component of hemoglobin, it carries oxygen to these tissues. Without it, the oxygen-starved muscles gradually become exhausted and the brain less focused. Symptoms of iron-deficiency anemia include pallor, fatigue, forgetfulness, depression, and shortness of breath.

As I detailed in Chapter Four, women are especially prone to iron deficiencies in part because of nature and in part because of the choices we make in diet style. Women lose 2–4 tablespoons of blood each month during menstruation, including 15–30 milligrams of iron. The contraceptive intrauterine device (IUD), by increasing menstrual blood loss, causes even greater iron loss; the birth control pill, by decreasing blood loss, helps retain iron.

Pregnancy further depletes supplies since the mother's blood supplies iron to the fetus. Of course, blood is lost during childbirth, too.

Chronic dieters, who avoid iron-rich meat and eggs out of concern over calories, and nutrition buffs, who avoid them out of concern over cholesterol and saturated fats, are the most likely to be deficient. Since at best only 30 percent of the iron taken in is absorbed, you must eat more than your body needs.

The RDA for women is:

age 19–50	15 milligrams
over 50	10 milligrams
pregnant or lactating	30 or 15 milligrams

Food sources include: meat, eggs, leafy greens, beets, kelp, dried beans, enriched cereals and whole grains, pumpkin and sesame seeds, and blackstrap molasses. The herbs yellow dock and dandelion root are additional sources. Cooking in iron pots provides small amounts of this important mineral in your diet, as well.

See Chapter Four for more on the virtues of meat and eggs.

Zinc

As a cofactor, zinc is essential for the conversion of the Omega 3 and 6 oils into prostaglandins. Zinc is essential for body protein synthesis, vitamin metabolism, proper growth, healing of wounds and burns, and development of the sex organs. It promotes the removal of harmful carbon dioxide and is directly involved in the body's metabolism of carbohydrates and energy. It forms part of the insulin component secreted by the pancreas. Zinc helps to enhance digestion, protects the body in stressful conditions, and plays an important role in many major metabolic reactions.

Zinc strengthens hair and nails, and helps keep skin unblemished. Deficiencies may cause disruption of menstruation.

The grabber's diet, which emphasizes processed foods, is likely to be zinc deficient since processing removes most zinc found naturally. Nutrition buffs who partake of the high-carbohydrate, low-fat diet popular in the 1980s are also likely to be deficient because the phytic acid in the grains they eat excessively interferes with zinc absorption.

The RDA for women is:

age 19 and over	12 milligrams
pregnant	15 milligrams
lactating	19 milligrams

Food sources include: oysters, clams, herring, blackstrap molasses, chicken, sesame and sunflower seeds, liver, whole bran, whole oatmeal, and wheat germ.

Manganese

Manganese is involved in female sex hormone production; the synthesis of vitamins B, C, and E; and the metabolism of protein, carbohydrates, and fat. Manganese food sources protect bones and ligaments and nourish the brain and nervous system. The mineral is important in the function of normal reproduction and the mammary glands. Animals that have lost their mothering instinct have been found to be manganese deficient.

Manganese is another mineral that appears to have a role in osteoporosis, loss of bone density. Paul Saltman, M.D., at the University of California at San Diego, evaluated blood and bone samples of women with severe osteoporosis and those with no sign of the disease. The osteoporotic women had a manganese level one quarter of the level of the other group. Manganese deficiency is also associated with disk problems and cartilage formation.

The mineral also helps regulate blood sugar levels so that long periods without food will not result in heavy sugar bingeing or a weakening low blood sugar attack. Diabetics, as well as schizophrenics and individuals prone to heart disease and rheumatoid arthritis, are often low in tissue blood levels of manganese.

If either iron or manganese is taken excessively, each may interfere with the other's absorption.

The RDA for women is 2.0–5.0 milligrams (more precise levels are not yet known).

Food sources include: sea vegetables, buckwheat, whole wheat, barley, whole brown rice, almonds, beans, peas, and pineapple.

Iodine

Iodine was one of the first minerals recognized as important to human health. It is the essential ingredient in the thyroid hormone thyroxine. This hormone controls metabolism, so that inadequate supplies can result in fatigue, overweight, and diminished sex drive.

Low levels of iodine can disrupt the breakdown of estrogen, resulting in excess estrogen and the problems it can cause. Deficiencies may also cause dry hair and skin.

Conversely, iodine has been shown helpful in fibrocystic breast disease and as an expectorant. In the levels found in cough syrups, however, it worsens acne.

The RDA for women is:

age 19 and over	150 micrograms
pregnant	175 micrograms
lactating	200 micrograms

Food sources include: sea vegetables, kelp, sea salt, herring, seafood, cod-liver oil, and vegetables grown in iodine-rich soil.

Copper

When everything is in balance, we have just a pinch of copper in our bodies. Yet it is essential for incorporating iron into hemoglobin; forming melanin for skin color and collagen for strong bones, joints, and connective tissue; and synthesizing neurotransmitters to carry impulses throughout the nervous system. Several enzymes need copper to build body tissue, and it contributes to fertility and completion of pregnancy. Copper aids in resistance to infection and retention of calcium in bones.

Copper is abundant in today's environment, so few women are technically deficient. More commonly, problems arise with imbalances in the delicate system of copper synthesis, resulting in biounavailable, unbound, and ultimately toxic copper.

Copper plumbing and cookware contribute to our copper load, as does the drinking water in some areas. The birth control pill tends to raise blood copper levels, and some experts believe copper may be absorbed from copper IUDs.

Our diet may contribute as well. Copper is an effective fungicide, so copper sulfate may be sprayed on fruits and vegetables. Soybeans and tofu, staples in the vegetarian diet, are naturally high in copper, as are oysters, calf and lamb liver, and regular tea.

Several physiological conditions affect copper usage and accumulation, the most important being the activity of the adrenal gland. When the adrenal gland malfunctions from stress—too much sugar or caffeine, alcohol, or tobacco—it causes ceruloplasmin production to slow down in the liver. Since about 95 percent of the copper in our blood is bound to ceruloplasmin, a prerequisite to copper use, without it unbound copper accumulates in the brain, liver, and other organs.

Zinc, which ideally should be present in a ratio of 8:1 with copper, helps prevent copper accumulation. However, with decreased consumption of zinc-rich meat and eggs and increased consumption of zinc-inhibiting sugars and grains, zinc deficiencies are common. In addition, sudden stress simultaneously raises blood copper levels and lowers blood zinc.

When copper is stored and not used, problems arise. High blood or tissue copper levels have been associated with:

- acne
- hair loss
- anemia
- rheumatoid arthritis
- premenstrual syndrome
- osteoporosis
- candidiasis (yeast infections)
- elevated estrogen levels
- decreased sexual function
- various nervous disorders, including depression, phobias, and schizophrenia

Blood tests can determine copper levels. Tissue mineral analysis (hair analysis) is still controversial, but its supporters argue it is the most effective way to measure a variety of heavy metals.

Several vitamins and minerals are known to lower copper levels, by binding with it to pull it out of storage or to carry it out of the body. These include vitamins B_6, C, folic acid, and niacin (B_3); and the minerals sulfur, molybdenum, iron, manganese, and zinc.

My diet plan outlined in the remaining chapters can help maintain the effective copper balance: it retains zinc-rich meat and eggs, monitors the copper-rich grains, and avoids the stressors sugars and caffeine.

The RDA for women is 2–3 milligrams (more specific levels have not been determined).

Food sources include: liver, kidneys, oysters, wheat germ, soybeans, mushrooms, blackstrap molasses, dried beans, and nuts.

PMS: A Deficiency Disorder?

There is a condition from which 70–90 percent of American women of childbearing age suffer . . . a condition that disrupts lives, causes recurring pain and suffering, and may even bring on violence and death . . . a condition that may have afflicted Queen Victoria and Mary Todd Lincoln . . . a condition for which there are no diagnostic tests, no clearly defined cause, no definitive cure . . . a condition called premenstrual syndrome, or just PMS.

What does PMS have to do with "female" minerals? Almost all of the minerals I have discussed (and a few others) have a role in various symptoms of PMS and, therefore, in therapy (see chart). In fact, nutritional imbalance and its integral role with hormonal imbalance may one day prove to be a key to unlocking this Pandora's box.

Nutrient Deficiencies and PMS

Nutrient	Status at menstruation	Effects
B_6 (pyridoxine)	deficient prior to	mood swings
calcium	lower prior to	muscle cramps, pelvic pain, bloating, nervousness
magnesium	may be lower prior to	cravings, mood swings, bloating, breast tenderness

Nutrient	Status at menstruation	Effects
zinc	may be deficient	headaches, irritability, depression or nervousness, cramps
iron	may be deficient	anemia, fatigue, weakness
potassium	may be deficient	fluid retention, headaches, tiredness
sodium	elevated	weight gain, bloating
copper	elevated	reduced adrenal activity, deficiencies in other minerals, mental depression
vitamin E	may be deficient	fluid retention, cramps, breast tenderness

While many women experience menstrual cramping, headaches, or low back pain during their period, PMS generally refers to the symptoms that occur 1–10 days prior to menstruation. These symptoms usually improve once menstruation begins. Most women have more than one symptom, but they usually experience the same cluster month after month.

Researcher Guy Abraham, M.D., has divided the symptoms into four subclasses, based on their most common groupings among women:[4]

PMS A (Anxiety) 65–75 percent of sufferers

- nervous tension
- mood swings

- irritability
- anxiety

Vitamin B$_6$ and magnesium are particularly helpful.

PMS H (Heavy) 50–65 percent of sufferers

- weight gain
- swelling of hands and feet
- abdominal bloating
- breast tenderness

Magnesium, vitamin B$_6$, and vitamin E may help relieve symptoms.

PMS C (Craving) 25–35 percent of sufferers

- headache
- craving for sweets or salty foods
- increased appetite
- dizziness or fainting spells
- fatigue

Vitamins B$_6$ and C, zinc, and GLA can help.

PMS D (Depression) 25–35 percent of sufferers

- depression
- forgetfulness
- crying
- confusion
- insomnia

Magnesium and essential fatty acids (EFAs) help some women.

The underlying cause or causes of PMS are not yet known. Several researchers, including Katharina Dalton of England, suspect an imbalance in the estrogen-progesterone ratio with excessive levels of estrogen. Furthermore, citing an apparent deficiency in EFAs among premenstrual women, some experts postulate that without adequate EFAs, the body will not produce enough prostaglandin E_1. This substance in turn has a controlling effect on the female hormone prolactin and complex interactions with steroids. Further supporting this theory is the known role that magnesium, zinc, and vitamins B_3, B_6, and C have in the conversion of EFA to PGE_1 (see Chapter Three).

Optimizing production of the prostaglandins from EFAs is central to the plan I recommend to my clients and describe in this book. In addition, the plan's emphasis on avoiding caffeine, sugar, and excess sodium is a built-in prescription for relief from PMS. Only when we choose health, when we take back control of our diets, will we control our hormones, not the other way around.

Super Female Foods

In Chapter Ten, I give a staples shopping list for foods that will help assure long-term health and fitness. However, because of their abundance of "female" minerals and other vitamins and minerals essential to every woman's good looks and health, I have designated some foods as Super Female Foods. Here's my list, along with the significant nutrients they contain:

- **Blackstrap molasses** (residue from sugar refining)—vitamins B_1, B_2, inositol, PABA; iron, calcium, magnesium, potassium, copper, chromium, molybdenum

- **Brewer's yeast** (dried yeast derived from brewing beer and ale)—vitamins B_1, B_2, B_3, B_6, B_{15}, folic acid, biotin, choline, PABA; iron, calcium, phosphorus, potassium, zinc, selenium, chromium. (Note: Moderation is essential with this one, since too much may encourage candida overgrowth.)

- **Broccoli**—vitamins A (beta carotene), C, folic acid; iron, calcium, selenium

- **Lentils**—vitamins B_1, B_6, pantothenic acid, folic acid, biotin, choline, inositol; iron, calcium, potassium

- **Sea vegetables**—vitamins A, B_1, B_2, B_3, B_{12}; calcium, magnesium, potassium, iodine, selenium, chromium, molybdenum, vanadium, lithium, silicon

- **Sesame seeds**—vitamins B_1, B_3, B_{15}, B_{17}; zinc, potassium, phosphorus, calcium, iron; EFAs

- **Sunflower seeds**—vitamins B_1, B_3, pantothenic acid, PABA; magnesium, potassium, zinc

- **Whole brown rice**—vitamins B_3, B_6, B_{15}, pantothenic acid, folic acid, biotin, choline; magnesium, manganese, selenium

Nutritional Treasures from the Sea

One item on the list of Super Female Foods is not yet familiar to many Americans, sea vegetables. Although they have an ancient past, sea vegetables are of particular interest today to women who want to ensure good health.

Sea vegetables have absorbed nutrients from the sea via not just their roots but also their leaves and stems. As the list above indicates, they are chock full of hard-to-find trace minerals, as well as the more common calcium and iron (10 times more than spinach). Here is a brief rundown on the more commonly available types, with suggestions for preparation:

- **Hijiki**—tastes a bit like licorice and looks like tangled black strings; contains 14 times the calcium in a glass of cow's milk. Rinse in cold water, then soak for 20 minutes. Hijiki can be added to soups or salads; it is delicious sautéed with carrots and fresh ginger.

- **Wakame**—a delicately flavored dark green leaf. Rinse in cold water, soak for 15 minutes. Add to soups, on top of fish, or in dressings.

- **Kombu**—a kelp with a sweet/salty flavor. It can be toasted in the oven for snacks, added to beans (aids digestion), or crumbled and sprinkled over fish, chicken, or rice dishes. Cut into strips, it can be added to soups.

- **Nori** (green laver or sea lettuce)—a nutty-tasting seaweed, high in B_{12} and A, that comes in sheets. It can be toasted and crumbled over vegetables, pasta, or fish. Or use it untoasted to wrap other foods.

- **Arame**—a taste and appearance similar to hijiki. Rinse in cool water, then soak for 10–15 minutes. It more than doubles in size, to be added to salads, soups, brown rice, and vegetables. Both hijiki and arame can also be sautéed for 2–3 minutes in oil.

- **Agar agar**—a seaweed that is sold in flake form to be used in place of gelatin for thickening puddings, molds, and mousses.

A Word About Supplements

Americans currently spend $2.5 billion annually on vitamin and mineral supplements. Clearly, millions of men and women think they are getting some value; the experts can't agree among themselves whether or not this is true.

For example, in early 1989, the National Research Council of the National Academy of Sciences issued a report in which they said, among other things, that while mineral supplements and multivitamins may not be harmful, there is no evidence they are helpful.

Supplements cannot and should not replace food. The delicate mineral balance needed for effective calcium utilization highlights the kind of chemistry nature provides—broccoli is not just a source of calcium, but also of beta carotene, vitamin C, iron, folic acid, and fiber. Imbalances can quickly arise if a single mineral is emphasized in supplements.

Nevertheless, most women will benefit from some supplementation. Environmental pollutants deplete nutrients from our bodies through the process of detoxification and elimination. Medications such as aspirin cancel out nutrients; birth control pills cause deficiencies of folic acid and vitamins B_6 and B_{12}. Topsoil depletion, food processing, and storage time decrease the levels of nutrients contained in foods.

Certain events in women's lives, such as pregnancy, lactation, and menopause, put such demands on our bodies that even the 3 percent of us who eat appropriate amounts from all the food groups are unlikely to meet our bodies' needs.

I would suggest that, given widespread deficiencies of zinc and magnesium and the need for these and other nutrients in the conversion of EFAs to the protective prostaglandins, women should take a multivitamin and mineral supplement containing: niacin (B_3), B_6, C, and E; antioxidant beta carotene; and minerals zinc, magnesium, and selenium.

Choosing especially nutrient-rich foods and supplementing key nutrients can help you feel and look better. If modern science will allow many of us to live longer than was thought possible just 50 or 100 years ago, then our responsibility to ourselves to make our later years healthy years is a great one. The following chapters outline my plan for us to take control of our health destiny.

TEN

What to Eat,

How to Heat

*You can't eat well and keep fit
if you don't shop well.*

—Adelle Davis, nutritionist

Label Reading: Worth the Effort

Since the average supermarket may contain over 20,000 items (with nearly 8,000 new food products entering the marketplace each year), label reading is a necessity. It is a fairly simple task to decode any food label once you understand the rules of the game.

The basic rule is that the Food and Drug Administration requires food manufacturers to list ingredients of greatest amount by descending order of weight. This means that if a "natural" or "lite" oatmeal cookie, for example, lists apple juice concentrate (fructose, a fruit sugar) as the first ingredient, then the cookie contains more concentrate than any other ingredient, including oats. Furthermore, the words *natural* and *lite* or *light* have no legal definition.

If a product carries a health claim, then additional information is also provided, such as calories; grams of protein, fat, and sodium; and vitamin and mineral content per serving. Many manufacturers are now listing dietary fiber and cholesterol grams for concerned consumers.

Fat Finding

Health experts agree that the high-fat diet Americans are eating (almost 40 percent of total calories) is linked to heart disease and some forms of cancer. An ideal low-fat menu plan should derive between 20 and 30 percent of calories from fat (the "good" fats). In my experience, reaching a happy medium of 25 percent calories from fat is a realistic and practical goal, when the fats include the essential fats.

Food labels, such as those on milk cartons, list fat by weight, not by calories. Our interest is in knowing the percentage of fat by calories, not by weight. Two percent milk may seem like a low-fat item, but in truth, it contains 36 percent fat.

In order to calculate percentage of fat by calories, remember that each gram of fat contains 9 calories, while each gram of protein or carbohydrate contains 4 calories. By calculating the number of fat calories and dividing by the total calories you can determine the percentage of fat calories in any food item from information on the label:

$$\frac{\text{Grams of fat per serving} \times 9}{\text{Total calories per serving}} = \text{percent fat}$$

(To find out the percentage of protein or carbohydrate calories, substitute 4 for the 9.)

Here is how the formula works. Let's say that, according to a package label, one serving (½ cup) of granola contains 9.8 grams of fat and 252 calories. Using the fat formula, the calculations would be:

$$\frac{9.8 \text{ grams of fat per serving} \times 9}{252} = 35 \text{ percent fat}$$

Thus, one serving of this particular brand of granola provides 35 percent fat calories per serving: an unwise food choice since it is 10 percent higher than the 25 percent recommendation.

Furthermore, the fat contained in foods that are canned, jarred, or packaged is usually the undesirable kind—either saturated (palm, palm kernel, or coconut oil) or damaged (processed vegetable oil, margarine, or shortening). Try to avoid these fat sources as much as possible by selecting preferred brand name products that contain essential or health oils (see below for complete listing).

Avoid luncheon meats, hot dogs, cold cuts, sausages, and other packaged meats. Not only do they often contain high levels of fat, but also they frequently have high levels of sodium and potentially hazardous additives.

The Guide to Reducing Dietary Fat, Appendix A, will help you figure out how many fat calories and fat grams to eat each day, based on a typical diet of 1,500, 2,000, and 2,500 calories. A listing of selected foods with their total calories, fat grams, and percentage of fat calories can be found in Appendix B to give you a better idea of hidden fats in your diet. The average woman should consume a total of 40–50 grams of fat per day.

For many of us, supermarket sleuthing is the only

way to avoid certain fats. When you learn to read the fine print, you will no doubt be in for some fat-filled surprises. Name brand products like Granny Goose bagel chips contain 9 grams of fat in one ounce. Pillsbury Original Flavor Microwave Popcorn contains 13 grams of fat in 3 cups, while Orville Redenbacher Microwave Popcorn comes in lower at 7 grams of fat in a 4-cup serving. A Roman Meal frozen whole grain waffle has 7 grams of fat, too. Armour's Chili with Beans (7½ ounces) packs a walloping 25 grams of fat!

Searching for Salt

It is unfortunate that all salt has gotten a bad reputation because of the detrimental effects of refined table salt. Table salt is an unbalanced salt excessively high in sodium chloride and stripped of its other essential trace minerals like magnesium, bromine, and sulfur. In proper mineral balance, natural salt is used by the body to cleanse mucous membranes, regulate body fluids, and normalize blood pressure. Not only is commercial table salt minerally unbalanced, it also contains a number of chemical additives, such as bleaches, conditioners, and anticaking agents, which are toxic to our systems. In fact, sodium chloride in an unadulterated pure form may very well be the most vital element contained in blood plasma.

When salt is refined and combined with other chemical additives, its metabolic functions are changed. Refined salt does not dissolve in the body; it hardens, leaving deposits in organs and tissue that can result in arterial plaque buildup. Any salt can be tested for its metabolic acceptability by adding 2 tablespoonfuls to a glass of plain water and letting it stand for a couple of hours. If no residue remains on the bottom of the glass, then the salt will dissolve in the fluids of the body as well. If residue remains, this signals unbalanced processed substances unfit for human consumption.

Sea salts are commercially available. Yet these salts can also be refined and may contain chemical pollutants from waste materials in our oceans.

Proper salt intake is essential, especially in summer and for athletes, because so much of the mineral leaves the body fluids via perspiration, tears, and urine.

The National Research Council suggests that 1,100–3,300 milligrams per day is a safe sodium intake for most adults. Many women, particularly those with high blood pressure or who retain fluid and bloat easily, need to watch salt intake more carefully. If you are one of these women, consider reducing your total sodium intake to about 1,500 milligrams (¾ teaspoon).

Since most of the salt in our diets comes from canned, bottled, frozen, and processed or fast foods, you will have to learn to decipher the various disguises of salt listed on food labels. When eating in fast-food restaurants, be aware that three pieces of Kentucky Fried Chicken contain 1,015 milligrams of sodium, McDonald's Big Mac delivers 962 milligrams, and its Egg McMuffin can add 914 milligrams to your diet. A Taco Bell Taco is one of your best bets at 79 milligrams. (Note that as in all fast foods, no matter what the sodium level, you may be getting too much of the wrong kinds of fats.)

To reduce high-sodium food items, try to avoid or cut down on the following:

- Snacks: chips, pretzels, crackers, dips
- Condiments: soy sauce, tamari, mustard, catsup, miso, capers, barbecue sauce, chili sauce, salad dressings, Worchestershire sauce, meat tenderizers, bouillon cubes, pickles, monosodium glutamate (MSG); also onion, celery, or garlic salts (powders are all right)

- Cured meats: hot dogs, luncheon meats, sausages, bacon
- Sauerkraut
- Cheese
- Canned fish and vegetables
- Self-rising white flour

Fortunately, many food items are now available with either "salt free" or "sodium restricted" brands, for which minimum standards have been set by the FDA. Later in this chapter I provide a listing of Healthy Foods in Convenient Packages.

Label ingredient listings that include baking powder, baking soda, sodium propionate (a mold inhibitor), sodium benzoate (a preservative), or other sodium derivatives (look for the -ate ending), no matter what their purpose, indicate high levels of sodium and are a warning signal. You can further cut down by choosing foods that are naturally low in sodium, including most fruits and vegetables, or that are labeled "very low sodium," which by law means a sodium content of 35 milligrams or less per serving.

There are several ways to add flavor without salt, some of which are given later in this chapter. I give additional tips in Chapter Twelve about using herbs, spices, flavor extracts, and alcohol in cooking to create taste without added salt.

Another way to control sodium at the table is by seasoning after cooking. Research has shown that salt added after cooking tastes stronger than when added before or during cooking. Remember, however, when you add salt that:

¼ teaspoon = 500 milligrams sodium
½ teaspoon = 1,000 milligrams
¾ teaspoon = 1,500 milligrams
1 teaspoon = 2,000 milligrams

Kelp powder, a seaweed powder, can be used in place of salt. Used in one-half the quantities of regular salt, kelp contains a potassium-sodium ratio of 3:1, which more resembles that contained in body fluids (5:1) than does salt (1:10,000).

Stalking Sugar

Most of our dietary intake of sugar (nearly 130 pounds per year) is tastefully hidden in packaged foods. Watch out for all sugar sources, and keep in mind that up to five different kinds of sugar can be listed for one product. It all adds up. The following names mean sugar to your body, no matter how you spell them:

- Juice concentrate: apple, pear, peach, pineapple
- Sucrose, dextrose, lactose, maltose, fructose
- Corn sweetener
- Barley or corn malt
- Syrup: corn, rice, maple, malt
- Sugar: invert, brown, raw
- Honey

Mannitol, sorbitol, and xylitol are "sugar"-free substitutes. They are actually sugar-based alcohols. Found mainly in sugar-free gums, candies, and baked goods for diabetics, they all contain both calories and carbohydrates and have been known to cause diarrhea in sensitive individuals.

Abandoning Aluminum

Label reading is also a way to prevent aluminum from entering your diet; your ultimate goal is to eliminate aluminum entirely from your food. Check ingredient listings for aluminum frequently used in salt, baking powder (unless label specifies nonaluminum baking powder), cake mixes, self-rising flour, processed American cheese, nondairy creamers, and pickled fruits and vegetables. Soft drinks (which are not recommended because of their bone-robbing phosphoric acid content) will add unwanted aluminum to your diet if they are packaged in aluminum cans. The same goes for many types of beer and mineral water.

Many waxed cardboard beverage containers, especially for juices, are lined with aluminum. The acidic fruits and vegetables leach the metal into the food.

Nonfood items, such as antacids, vaginal douches, and antidiarrhetics, can also contain this heavy metal. Substitute products without aluminum.

The Staples Kitchen of the 1990s: Confessions of a Fast-food Nutritionist

Fast-food nutrition is no longer a contradiction in terms. Over the years I have discovered many shortcuts to wholesome foods without shortchanging nutrition. Like so many women, I am constantly on the go and have had to translate the concerns of the chronic dieter, nutrition buff, and grabber into fit but fast foods.

It is also true that, by nature, I really don't like to

cook . . . but I do love to eat, so healthy convenience foods are doubly important to me. I also favor eating organically grown produce and meats and poultry raised without artificial hormones or antibiotics. Based on my own hectic life-style and desire to eat "safe" foods, I have developed a standard list of food staples that I shop for whether at home or on the road.

I am providing my list with the brand names that I personally use. Many of these foods can currently be found in a well-stocked "health food" section of your supermarket or at your natural food store or food cooperative. Since increasing numbers of food retailers are concerned about the consumer's rising interest in pesticide- and preservative-free food, you may find your local store manager receptive to your suggestions of products to stock.

This list features packaged, jarred, or canned foods. A complete shopping list for total nutrition appears later in this chapter.

Healthy Foods in Convenient Packages

Dairy Products
Continental, Colombo, Weight Watcher's, and Dannon fat-free yogurts

Star's frozen yogurt (I prefer the fruit-juice sweetened to the fructose-honey sweetened varieties)

Altadena dry curd cottage cheese

Calabro 100 percent skim milk ricotta cheese

Lifetime Swiss, mozzarella, mild cheddar, and Monterey Jack. The Lifetime natural part-skim-milk cheeses are reduced at least 50 percent in fat calories and salt, yet contain at least 30 percent

more calcium than commercial varieties. They
are great for melting on a rice cake with a touch
of mustard, caraway seeds, or hot pepper sauce.

Fast Fixes (side dishes, appetizers, snacks)
Arrowhead Mills quick brown rice
Barbara's instant mashed potatoes
Ancient Harvest quinoa elbow pasta
Energy Food Factory Poprice (baked brown rice
    snack)
Fantastic Foods Fantastic Falafel or Tabouli
Lundberg RizCous (like couscous, only rice) Cajun
    or French country herb style
Nile Spice couscous salad mix, basmati rice, and red
    lentils
Carmel Kosher potato pancake or kugel mixes
Deep Roots side dishes
Health Valley lentil pilaf, amaranth pilaf, jalapeno
    bean dip, onion bean dip, taco dip, taco sauce
Jaclyn's breaded veggies (mushrooms or cauliflower)
Rice Tech Pastariso pastas (100% rice)
Organ rye, rice and millet pastas
Vita-spelt whole spelt pasta

Canned Foods
Water-packed tuna or salmon
3 Diamond mackerel fillets (drain well and rinse
    under running water)
Lillie's skinless and boneless sardines, packed in
    water
Water chestnuts
Chung King Chinese vegetables
Ortega chilies
Black pitted olives (rinse under running water)

Soups
Hain turkey rice, minestrone, vegetable chicken,
   Italian vegetable, Italian vege-pasta
Health Valley split pea
Pritikin chicken broth, chicken gumbo

Frozen Foods
Northwest Natural Salmon Medallions
Health Valley turkey or chicken wieners (nitrate free)
Shelton's turkey breakfast sausage (nitrate free)
Bounty of the Sea tuna franks
Cascadian Farms strawberries or raspberries, green
   beans or cauliflower (organic)

Cereals
American Prairie hot and cold cereals (organic)
Kolln Oat Bran Crunch
Kashi 5 Bran Instant Cereal
Lundberg creamy rice (organic)
Pocono cream of buckwheat
Spicer's Wheatsnacks. Spicer's snacks are a high-fiber
   (6 grams per 1½ ounces) food. The peanut, chocolate (processed without butterfat or caffeine),
   barbecue, and sour cream and onion are perfect
   for "grazing." Any Spicer's snack can be used as
   a total meal replacement when you just don't
   have time to eat. Look for Spicer's snacks at your
   health food, discount, or drug store.

Breads, Crackers, Tortillas, and Taco Shells
Ponce sourdough bread
Baldwin Hills sourdough rye or whole wheat bread
Shelburne Farms sourdough bread
Lundberg rice cakes (organic)

Westbrae brown rice wafers
Snackcracks organic brown rice crackers
Bran A Crisp
Fiber Rich bran crackers
Garden of Eatin blue corn tortillas and corn tortillas
   (organic)
Fiber Crisp rye crackers
Ry Vita
Lifestream Wheat and Rye Krispbread (organic)
Wasa Crispbread hearty and golden rye
Finn crisp rye
Kavli rye
Nejaimes Lavasch (Armenian crackerbread)
Little Bear blue corn and corn taco shells (organic)
Sprout Muffins (Sprout Delights Bakery in Miami,
   FL)

Snacks
Nuts, unshelled: almonds, walnuts, filberts, and pea-
   nuts
Seeds: sunflower, sesame, and pumpkin
Ralph's low-salt Bavarian pretzels
Popcorn (airpopped)
Arrowhead Mills Deaf Smith peanut butter (organic)
The Bean Chip (salted or unsalted)
Westbrae almond butter
Arrowhead Mills sesame tahini (organic)

Condiments
Spectrum canola mayonnaise
Dijon salt-free mustard
Westbrae sugar-free Unketchup
Enrico's spaghetti sauce with mushrooms
Tree of Life no-salt added pasta sauce or salsa
   (organic)

New England organic dill pickles (no salt)
Rosarita enchilada sauce
Balsamic or raspberry vinegar
Vanilla extract
Variety of dried herbs and nonirradiated spices: garlic
    powder, onion powder, dill, cumin, parsley,
    basil, cinnamon, oregano, rosemary

Beverages
Sparkling mineral waters
Filtered water
Water with lemon or lime
Frey wines (organic)
Domaine de la Busque wines (organic)
Assorted herbal teas
Pau d'Arco or taheebo herb tea (thought by some to
    be beneficial to candida sufferers)
Altura coffee (organic). I keep this on hand for guests,
    since I don't drink coffee.
Bio Drink or Kotobuki (made by Apollo Interna-
    tional). This is a fermented concentrated liquid
    made from natural apple cider vinegar and brown
    rice vinegar. It is a great substitute for alcohol,
    coffee, or tea, if candida overgrowth is not a prob-
    lem. Bio Drink helps establish the proper pH
    balance in the body and assists in calcium and
    iron absorption. It comes in single servings and
    can be combined with 8–10 ounces of cold or hot
    water. Available in health food stores.

Sweet Treats
Rice Dream carob-coated bars (yes, there is coconut
    oil in the coating, but also lecithin, which is a fat
    emulsifier; it's my only cheat)
Le Sorbet

Gone Bananas carob-coated bananas frozen with peanuts

Lifestream Essene fruit cake, raisin, pumpernickel-rye, seed, multigrain, cinnamon-date, rye seed, and muffins (great toasted plain)

Fearn carob or banana cake mixes

A Note About Pesticides and Food Irradiation

While taste, convenience, and nutrition are important factors in selecting foods, women are also concerned about the overuse of pesticides in America's food supply. The organization Mothers and Others for Pesticides Limits, a project of the Natural Resources Defense Council, has brought the safe food fight to the forefront.

I urge you to protect yourself and your family by looking for organic produce (check your local health food store or food cooperative), buying domestically grown fruits and vegetables in season (imported produce can contain pesticides banned in the U.S.), and growing your own foods in gardens or planter boxes.

Exposing foods to radiation leaves very dangerous residues. Food and Water can provide you with information on what you can do to stop radiation-exposed food. Call 1-800-EAT-SAFE.

I have also been concerned about the growing number of both chemicals and parasites in America's food supply for many years. The use of insecticides, fungicides, and weed killers is over double that of 20 years ago—about 800 million pounds of these chemicals per year.

Below is the detoxifying cleansing bath that I use for all kinds of foods: fruits, vegetables, beef, poultry, eggs, fish, and shellfish. It has been used successfully by my patients for over 12 years.

1. Use ½ teaspoon Clorox bleach to 1 gallon of water, obtained from your usual source. Only the Clorox brand will work, so do not substitute any other product.

2. Place the foods to be treated into the bath according to the chart below. Make a separate bath for each group.

3. Remove foods from the Clorox bath and place in clear water for 10 minutes. Dry all foods thoroughly and store.

Food Cleansing Schedule

Food group	Treatment time
Vegetables, leafy	15 minutes
Vegetables, root, thick-skinned, or fibrous	30 minutes
Fruits, thin-skinned berries, peaches, apricots, plums	15 minutes
Fruits, thick-skinned such as apples, citrus, and bananas	30 minutes
Chicken, fish, meats, eggs	20 minutes

Note: Meats can be thawed in a Clorox bath. The timing is about 20 minutes for a weight of 2 to 5 pounds. Frozen turkey or chicken should remain in the Clorox bath until thawed. Ground meats, of course, cannot undergo this process.

ALERT: If you suspect your food has been irradiated, then first clean food with a solution of 2 tablespoons of baking soda to 1 gallon of water and leave for 20 minutes. Then place in clear water for 10 minutes. Continue with Clorox bath program as outlined. Most chicken and potatoes are now irradiated.

The Complete Kitchen of the 1990s: A Guide to Stocking and Serving Portions

Throughout this book, I have made suggestions for foods to eat or to avoid. Here it is, all put together to give you a guide to selecting foods that will help you avoid deficiencies, especially zinc, calcium, magnesium, iron, phosphorus, potassium, and the B vitamins.

Essential and Healthy Fats

Choose from a variety of healthy and essential fat sources. Look for the words *100 percent expeller-pressed* on the label. Spectrum Naturals make a wide variety of healthful oils and are strong advocates of educating the consumer on the importance of oils in the diet. One to two tablespoons of oil a day, either as pure oil or from any of the food sources listed below, is all it takes for healthy skin, hair, and nails, and good reproductive health. Even cholesterol management is enhanced by using the right cooking oils.

Oils to choose from include: safflower, sunflower, corn, sesame, pumpkin seed, peanut, avocado, olive, canola, hazelnut, walnut, flaxseed, rice bran, almond, high-oleic safflower, and high-oleic sunflower.

Each food source listed below is broken down to equal the equivalent of one teaspoon of oil (i.e., a tablespoon of pumpkin seeds or of mayonnaise equals one teaspoon of pure oil).

Nuts (all raw or home toasted in oven)	
Nut	*Amount*
Almonds	7
Brazil nuts	2 medium

Nut	Amount
Cashews	4–5
Hazelnuts (filberts)	5
Macadamia nuts	3
Pecans	5 halves
Pine nuts (pignolias)	1 tablespoon
Pistachios	15
Walnuts	4 halves
Seeds (raw or home toasted, 1 tablespoon): pumpkin, sunflower, squash, and sesame, among others	
Mayonnaise (expeller-pressed or canola oil): 1 tablespoon	

Many of the natural oils have a distinct flavor, making some better for salads, others for sautéeing. This chart will help you select the best oil for each method.

Oil Selection by Cooking Method

Oil	Cooking	Baking	Frying	Sautéeing	Sauces	Salads
Canola	X	X	X	X		X
Corn						X
Olive, pure	X			X	X	X
Olive, extra virgin	X			X	X	X
Peanut	X			X	X	
High-oleic safflower	X	X	X			X
Regular safflower	X	X				X

Oil	Cooking	Baking	Frying	Sautéeing	Sauces	Salads
Sesame	X	X		X	X	X
High-oleic sunflower	X	X	X			

Vegetables

A portion equals ½ cup cooked or 1 cup raw, unless otherwise indicated. Of special interest to women are calcium-rich vegetables like bok choy, broccoli, kale, and sea vegetables. Try to eat colorfully for all-around nutrition: orange and yellow foods feature vitamins A and C; red and blue foods (like beets and seaweeds) give us iron; green foods highlight magnesium and vitamin A. They are all valuable sources of dietary fiber; each serving contains between 2 and 3 grams of fiber. At least four colorful servings of vegetables and fruits are suggested daily. *Note:* Frequent intake of greens from beets, dandelion, mustard, turnips, as well as spinach and sorrel, should be limited because of the calcium-inhibiting effects of oxalic acid.

Artichoke (½ large, cooked)

Asparagus

Beans (both green and yellow)

Beets

Bok choy (Chinese chard or white mustard cabbage)

Broccoli

Brussels sprouts

Cabbage

Carrots

Carrot juice (¼ cup or 2 fluid ounces)

Cauliflower

Celery

Cilantro (coriander or Chinese parsley)

Chicory

Chilies

Chinese cabbage (napa)

Cucumber

Daikon (long white radish)

Eggplant

Endive

Escarole

Garlic

Greens (collard, radicchio, arugula, mache)

Jerusalem artichoke (sunchoke)

Jicama

Kale

Lettuce (romaine, bibb, Boston)

Mushrooms

Okra

Onions

Parsley

Peppers (all colors)

Radishes

Rutabaga

Snow peas (Chinese pea pods)

Spinach

Sprouts (alfalfa, radish, mung bean, clover, adzuki)

Squash (yellow or crookneck, Italian or zucchini, spaghetti, chayote)

Tomatoes

Vegetable juice (½ cup)

Watercress

Water chestnuts (6 whole)

Sea vegetables: Eden has the widest variety of packaged sea vegetables available, including nori, hijiki, kombu, and arame. Particularly rich in calcium and iron, they can be used in soups, as edible garnishes, or as side dishes. Nutrient information and some suggested cooking tips are included in Chapter Nine.

Fruits

Since many women overdo fruits in the mistaken belief that because they are natural they can be eaten without limits, suggested portions are indicated to help you monitor your intake. Each portion contains about 2 grams of fiber. Remember at least four servings of fruits and vegetables are recommended daily. If candida is out of control, the sugar from fruits should be substantially reduced (just one fruit a day) or even temporarily avoided. Keep in mind that eating the fresh fruit itself, rather than in juice form, provides dietary fiber and is more filling. The fruits listed here are all fresh, sundried, or packed without sugar or syrup.

Fruit	*Serving portion*
Apple	1 small (2-inch diameter)
Apple butter (sugar free)	2 tablespoons
Apple juice or cider	⅓ cup
Applesauce (unsweetened)	½ cup
Apricots (fresh)	2 medium
Apricots (dried)	4 halves
Banana	½ small
Berries: boysenberries, blackberries, blueberries, raspberries	½ cup
Cantaloupe	¼ (6-inch diameter)
Cherries	10 large
Dates	2
Figs (fresh)	1 large
Figs (dried)	1 small
Fruit cocktail (canned in juice)	½ cup

Fruit	Serving portion
Fruit preserves and spreads (sugar free)	2 tablespoons
Grapefruit	½ small
Grapefruit juice	½ cup
Grapes	12
Grape juice	¼ cup
Honeydew melon	⅛ (7-inch diameter)
Mandarin oranges (canned)	¾ cup
Kiwi	1 medium
Mango	½ small
Nectarine	1 small
Orange	1 small
Orange juice (any style)	½ cup
Papaya	¾ cup
Peach	1 medium
Pear	1 small
Persimmon	1 medium
Pineapple	½ cup
Pineapple juice	⅓ cup
Plums	2 medium
Prunes	2 medium
Prune juice	¼ cup
Raisins	2 tablespoons
Strawberries	¾ cup
Tangerine	1 large
Watermelon	1 cup

Complex Carbohydrates

Vary your choices of complex carbohydrates for the best results. Gluten-based cereals from whole wheat, rye, oats, and barley should be taken in moderation; healthy alternatives include brown rice, millet, and buckwheat groats. Whole unprocessed grains, enriched cereals, and legumes are good iron sources. The yellow-orange starchy vegetables (like sweet potatoes) are vitamin A powerhouses. All add dietary fiber to your diet. Specifically, you get about 2 grams of fiber per serving from whole grain breads and crackers. Unrefined cereals and starchy vegetables provide about 3 grams of fiber per serving. Dried peas, beans, and lentils average from 4 to 8 grams of fiber per serving.

All yellow and orange vegetables, such as carrots, squash, yams, and sweet potatoes, are good beta carotene sources. In order to absorb the vitamin A in this preform, the body must first break down the beta carotene from the plant tissue. These vegetables must be prepared in such a way that the cell membrane is ruptured. Mashing, steaming, and shredding are the best ways to assure maximum absorption from the beta carotene–rich vegetables. Three or more servings per day are suggested.

Starchy Vegetables	Serving portion
Chestnuts, roasted	4 large or 6 small
Corn (on the cob)	1 (4 inches long)
Corn (cooked)	⅓ cup
Parsnips	1 small
Peas (fresh)	¾ cup
Potatoes (sweet, yam)	¼ cup
Potatoes, white (baked or boiled)	1 small

Starchy Vegetables	Serving portion
Potatoes, white (mashed)	½ cup
Pumpkin	¾ cup
Rutabaga	1 small
Squash (winter, acorn, butternut, buttercup)	½ cup
Succotash	½ cup

Breads

Bagel, whole wheat	½ small
Bread, rye, pumpernickel, whole wheat	1 slice
Breadsticks	4 (7 inches long)
Bun, hamburger or hot dog	½
Croutons	½ cup
English muffin	½
Pancakes	2 (3-inch diameter)
Pita bread	½ (6-inch pocket)
Rice cakes	2
Roll	1 (2-inch diameter)

Cereals and Grains

Barley (cooked)	½ cup
Bran flakes	½ cup
Bran (unprocessed rice or wheat)	⅓ cup
Buckwheat groats (kasha) (cooked)	⅓ cup
Cornmeal (cooked)	½ cup
Couscous	⅓ cup
Cream of rice (cooked)	½ cup
Grapenuts	¼ cup
Grits (cooked)	½ cup

Starchy Vegetables	Serving portion
Millet (cooked)	½ cup
Oatmeal	½ cup
Popcorn	3 cups
Puffed rice, wheat, millet, or oats	1½ cups
Rice (brown, cooked)	⅓ cup
Rice (wild, cooked)	½ cup
Shredded wheat biscuit	1 large
Tapioca	2 tablespoons
Wheatena (cooked)	½ cup
Wheat germ	1 ounce or 3 table-spoons

Crackers

Matzoh, whole wheat	½ (6 × 4 inches)
Pretzels, whole grain	1 large
Rice wafers, brown rice (Westbrae)	4
Rye crispbread crackers (Wasa)	1½ crackers
Wheat crackers, whole wheat (Ak-Mak)	4 crackers
(Health Valley)	13 crackers

Flours

Arrowroot	2 tablespoons
Buckwheat	3 tablespoons
Cornmeal	3 tablespoons
Cornstarch	2 tablespoons
Potato flour	2½ tablespoons
Rice flour	3 tablespoons
Soya powder	3 tablespoons
Whole wheat	3 tablespoons

Legumes

Beans, dried (cooked) lima, navy, pinto, kidney, garbanzos, black	½ cup
Beans, baked plain	½ cup
Lentils, dried (cooked)	½ cup
Peas, dried (cooked)	½ cup

Pasta

Noodles, macaroni, spaghetti (cooked)	½ cup
Noodles, rice (cooked)	½ cup
Noodles, whole wheat (cooked)	½ cup
Pasta, whole wheat (cooked)	½ cup

Protein

Include at least two 3-ounce servings of lean beef, fish, poultry, and other foods high in protein each day, including up to 4 eggs per week. Each food source is broken down to equal the equivalent of 1 ounce (cooked weight) of beef, fish, or poultry.

Remember, beef is graded in three categories. Select is the leanest grade, at 8 percent fat by weight, followed by Choice at 11 percent fat, then Prime at 14 percent fat. Make your choices from the Select grade whenever possible.

Soybeans are listed in the protein group because, although they are technically a legume, their fat content (30 percent of total calories) more nearly resembles that of a protein food. They are also used in vegetarian diets as a meat substitute.

Shelton Farms, Harmony Farms, Foster Farms, and

Young's Farm, commercial farm brands carried in natural food stores, offer organically raised chickens and turkeys. Lean and Free can send hormone- and antibiotic-free beef via mail order throughout the country (1-800-383-BEEF). Other sources for organic beef are Country B3R Meats (based in Childress, Texas) and Coleman Natural Beef (based in Denver, Colorado).

Food source	Serving portion
Cheese	
Lifetime Swiss, mozzarella, mild cheddar and Monterey Jack	1 ounce
Dry curd, skimmed, 1 percent or less low-fat cottage cheese	2 ounces
Egg, free-range, fertile	1
Fish and Seafood	
Salmon, halibut, perch, sole	1 ounce
Mussels, oysters, clams, shrimp, scallops	5 small
Lobster, calamari	1 ounce
Anchovies (well rinsed)	9 fillets
Sardines	3 medium
Canned salmon, tuna, crab	2 ounces
Meat and Poultry	
Poultry: white meat of skinned turkey and skinned chicken	1 ounce
Beef: lean—flank, top loin, ground tip, eye of round, sirloin, tenderloin	1 ounce
Lamb: leg, loin, rib	1 ounce
Veal: shoulder, rib, loin	1 ounce
Soybeans, tofu, and tempeh	1 ounce

Dairy

Choose two servings a day from this group. If you have difficulty digesting milk sugar (lactose intolerance is especially common among blacks, Mexicans, Asians, and Jews of Eastern European descent), consuming dairy products in which the lactose has been converted into lactic acid may be helpful. Yogurt and other fermented dairy products like kefir, buttermilk, or acidophilus milk are usually better tolerated by the lactose intolerant. You can also purchase enzymes under the trade name Lact-Aid to use in regular milk. You may need calcium supplements, but remember that there are other dietary sources of calcium besides dairy products. Removing the inhibitors from your diet will help you make the most of the calcium you do get, whatever the source.

Dairy	Serving portion
Milk: nonfat cow's milk, buttermilk, acidophilus milk, goat's milk	1 cup
Yogurt: nonfat cow's milk, plain; goat's milk yogurt, plain; kefir	1 cup
Soya powder (milk substitute)	3 tablespoons

How to Heat

Stir Sautéeing

Cook foods in small amounts of liquid or oil (water, peanut oil, canola oil, virgin olive oil, vegetable broth, or defatted chicken broth) at medium heat. Do not use polyunsaturated vegetable oils such as safflower or corn, which are extremely heat sensitive.

Steaming

Steaming preserves nutrients, color, and texture, and accentuates flavor while keeping in moisture. Cook over boiling water in a steamer pot, stainless steel folding basket, or Chinese-style tiered bamboo steamer. The leftover liquid can be used for soups or stir sautéeing.

When cooking highly concentrated carbohydrate foods such as sweet potatoes and yams, steam instead of baking. The baking temperatures precipitate the natural sugar into a caramelized substance, changing the complex carbohydrate into a simple sugar.

Broiling

Cook in a broiler with overhead direct heat. Keep the oven door open. Nutrients are destroyed when the oven door is closed because the food dehydrates when surrounded by dry heat.

Toasting

Cook in the oven at baking temperatures below 300 degrees. Seeds and nuts should be "home toasted." Low-level heating deactivates the enzyme inhibitors. Heating above 300 degrees, common in commercial roasting practices, changes the oil from the natural cis-form to the damaged trans-form.

Baking

Cook in covered dishes with minimum liquid to retain moistness.

Microwave

Microwave cooking heats the food by friction of the food's molecules. This is opposite to other cooking methods, in which the outside air surrounding the food must first be heated before the food begins to cook.

Cooking in a microwave does not make the food radioactive, despite the common misconception. Microwave cooking may even protect vitamins and minerals better than conventional methods, but care must be taken with certain foods. Because microwaves do not cook uniformly, rotating meats such as chicken and pork is necessary to protect against salmonella in the chicken and trichina in the pork.

Food prepared in a microwave may not be as visually appealing or appetizing because it does not brown after cooking. Convection microwave ovens or ovens with special browning features can achieve a more finished food look.

How Not to Heat

Frying

Frying is all too common in coffee shops and restaurants, as well as in the preparation of popular snack foods, such as doughnuts, potato chips, and many bakery products. Tasty as these foods are, overheating of polyunsaturated oils brings on oxidation of the oils and produces more free radicals than overheating of saturated fats; free radicals damage cells and may be the cause of aging. These foods should carry the Surgeon General's warning! Frying meat, fish, or chicken also makes the protein bond indigestible.

When palm or coconut oil is used for frying, there are many fewer free radicals formed because these oils are saturated. Too much of the saturated oils present another problem, though, because their presence can block the natural cis-linoleic acid from transforming to the vital GLA. Plus, harmful toxins that have been associated with cancer are produced no matter what source of fat is used when it is heated at high temperatures (350 degrees) or reheated with the same oil source. When you do fry, do not reheat the oil; throw it out.

Browning, Charring, or Charcoal Grilling

The oxidative reaction of charcoal grilling (a combination of browning and charring) is toxic and can be carcinogenic. Further, food soaks up added chemicals, including benzopyrenes, from the charcoal briquettes. One piece of barbecued meat may be the carcinogenic equivalent of 60 cigarettes. Charcoal broiling should be avoided, but if you do grill, use a raised wire grill to lessen contact of the meat with the charcoal, cook 4–6 inches away from the heat source, cut off any burned, charred, or blackened portions of meat, or better yet, choose quick-cooking fish, rather than meat, to grill.

Gas grilling—with adequate ventilation—is acceptable if there is no sensitivity to hydrocarbons, the toxic byproducts of gas combustion.

Pressure Cooking

Don't. The temperatures are too high and destroy vitamins. This method is suitable, however, for canning foods at home.

Electric Versus Gas?

For those who are environmentally sensitive, it is better to use electric rather than gas ranges and ovens for your cooking needs. The pilot lights and burners on gas ranges can release low levels of carbon monoxide and nitrous dioxide that often go undetected because they are invisible and odorless. Undiagnosable psychiatric conditions have even been traced to natural gas leakages. Symptoms such as dizziness, headache, chronic fatigue, confusion, insomnia, and respiratory problems can have their roots in unrecognized gas emissions.

If you suspect that you may be suffering from "indoor pollution," have your local gas company come to your house and check for a gas leak.

There are many other individuals who feel that the electromagnetic energy of food is disturbed with electric ranges and so prefer gas with proper ventilation.

Pots and Pans to Choose

1. Stainless steel—heavy-gauge stainless steel waterless cookware cooks food in a vacuum seal in its own juices. This is more expensive than the regular stainless, which is also recommended. Stainless steel, by the way, unless it is a high-gauge product, can be combined with an undesirable copper or aluminum base (see below).

2. Enamel cookware.

3. Corning Ware.

4. Glass and Pyrex—because glass and Pyrex let in light, they may allow small amounts of light-sensitive riboflavin to be depleted. Other items are unaffected. Amber-tinted glass is now available and is a better choice than clear glass.

5. Iron pots—the extra iron picked up from cooking is

good for you. When spaghetti sauce, for example, is cooked in iron pots, it contains six times more iron than when made in ceramic cookware.

Baking equipment should be heavy-duty tin or black steel. Glass, stainless steel bowls, cling-free plastic wrap, or plastic bags (the kind used in the produce section of the supermarket) are best for food storage and freezing. There is also a hypoallergenic cellophane bag now available at health food stores for more sensitive individuals. The above-mentioned materials do not dissolve into the food.

What Not to Choose

1. Aluminum cookware. Aluminum-proof the kitchen—as I have indicated, aluminum hampers the body's utilization of calcium, magnesium, and phosphorus, as well as vitamin A. Impaired memory and motor coordination, as well as Alzheimer's disease and osteoporosis, have been linked to systemic aluminum toxicity.

Check all pots, pans, steamers, measuring cups, spoons, bread pans, and cookie sheets. Even items made of aluminum layered between steel can "aluminate" food. These items can all be safely replaced by Pyrex or dairy tin (an old-fashioned baking material). An easy way to check for aluminum is with a small magnet; it will not stick to aluminum.

No food or drink, especially acidic foods that are tomato-based, should be cooked or covered in aluminum or aluminum foil. Instead of foil, use parchment paper in cooking and reheating. It is available in most health food stores and is excellent for retaining flavor because the food cooks in its own juice. Made from wood pulp, it is a healthy alternative to metals and plastics. Ideal for vegetables and fish (as New Orleans cooks have known for years), parchment paper can be used for baking and poaching. The food is placed on top of a moistened parchment sheet, then the corners are gathered up and tied securely.

2. Avoid unlined copper pots and pans—copper can contaminate acidic food and destroy vitamin C; it is also antagonistic to zinc. Brass containers are usually made with copper, so do not store food in them.

3. Replace or give a Clorox bath to wooden cutting and chopping boards—bacteria can live in the cracks of wooden blocks. Use a Lucite chopping board, or give your wooden board a Clorox rinse (use approximately 10 drops of Clorox bleach to a quart of water).

4. Throw out cracked dishes—again, bacteria can live in the cracks of cups and plates. These bacteria will mix with hot beverages or foods, creating digestive problems.

Just a Note About Life in the Great Outdoors

When camping out, remember to take extra care with certain foods. Ground meat is more subject to oxidation than whole meat. Cook it as soon as possible.

Do not drink water from streams and lakes, because many are contaminated with a protozoa called *Giardia lamblia*, the most frequent cause of waterborne illness in the country today. This amoeba-like one-celled animal can cause chronic diarrhea and has been implicated in chronic fatigue syndrome, allergy, and malabsorption. It makes its home in the upper gastrointestinal tract and gallbladder. Boil all questionable water for at least 10 minutes at a rolling boil.

ELEVEN

A Guide for

Dining Out

A cheerful heart hath a continual feast.

—Proverbs 15:15

Did you know that, in 1987, almost half of all Americans ate out more than once a day, and 92 percent ate out on a regular basis? These statistics were reported in *The Surgeon General's Report on Nutrition and Health*, a 750-page report released in 1988. Based on eating trends in the 1980s, this means that eating out will be more common than eating in, in the 1990s.

There are some basic food considerations to keep in mind when dining out. First, look for foods that feature the essential or healthy fats. Choose cuisines that use olive oil (Italian, Greek, Spanish, and in some cases, French). Some Japanese and Chinese dishes use either sesame or peanut oil for stir frying. Even carefully chosen Mexican dishes are good nutritional choices; guacamole features the heart-protecting monounsaturated fats and can be used as an appetizer or topping, instead of sour cream or cheese.

Keep in mind that the majority of undesirable saturated and damaged fats, salts, and sugars are hidden in sauces and dressings. Ask for all sauces and dressings on the side. Dip your fork into the dressing before it goes into the salad to control total fat intake. Pass over creamed sauces in favor of wine-based sauces, such as coq au vin (chicken cooked in red wine sauce). Likewise, try to avoid creamed soups in favor of tomato-based, vegetable, or bean soups. Choose Manhattan instead of New England clam chowder, for example.

Avoid unwanted fats by ordering seafood, beef, and poultry broiled, poached, or grilled and ask that no fat be used for basting during cooking.

Eliminate tuna, shrimp, chicken, and egg salads from your diet when eating out because they are usually loaded with too much commercial mayonnaise. Mayonnaise is actually a processed food containing heat-treated and partially hydrogenated soybean oil. At home you can use brands such as Spectrum canola mayonnaise or make it yourself from expeller-pressed oils.

When eating out, watch salad bar offerings like cole slaw, potato salad, and pasta salads, which can also be loaded with mayonnaise. Instead of mayonnaise- (or sour cream-) based dips, order guacamole, hummus (chick pea spread), or Mexican salsas. "Lemonize" these dips by lacing them with lemon or lime to further cut the amount of fat. For sandwiches, substitute mustard and add healthy, tasty items like lettuce, tomato, and onion.

In the bread department, best bets are whole wheat, rye, or sourdough bread and rolls. Prebuttered rolls, toast, and croissants (at 2–3 teaspoons of baked-in butter per croissant) should be limited. While butter is a more healthful choice than margarine, it still should be taken in moderation. One pat of butter per meal, on a baked potato, for example, is usually reasonable. Eliminate margarine entirely. Ordering onions, chives, leeks, and garlic with meals adds both taste and fat-fighting benefits.

You should basically avoid all fried foods, especially those with breading; the bread coating increases fat absorption, giving breaded, fried chicken and fish a higher fat content than a juicy hamburger. Other fried no-nos include tortilla chips, potato skins, Chinese egg or spring rolls, shrimp or vegetable tempura, and french fries. At home, you can make your own fries by coating sliced potatoes with a drop of canola or olive oil and then baking them in the oven.

Starting your meal with a cup or bowl of hot soup can actually help you cut calories, while adding valuable nutrients. A study at St. Luke's–Roosevelt Hospital, New York, found that when a group started its meal with soup, for every calorie the soup added to the meals, two fewer calories were eaten with the entree. The researchers believe that the soup moves into the small intestine more quickly than solid food, so triggers satiety receptors faster. See below for some nutritious choices.

A Note About Seafood

With the growing pollution of our rivers, streams, and oceans, there is some cause for concern about the fish and seafood that inhabit these waters. Not enough is known about the long-term effects of consuming contaminated fish and shellfish. At this time, however, experts agree with Clyde Dawe, M.D., a Harvard Medical School researcher who has studied the problem for more than 25 years, "People should not be so scared that they stop eating fish."[1]

However, it does pay to be a wise consumer of fish and shellfish. The experts recommend the following:

- Eat a variety of seafood to lessen your contamination from any one source.

- Cook seafood thoroughly. Avoid all raw fish or shell-fish.

- Ask about the source of the fish you purchase. Most fish is caught beyond three miles from the coastal waters, safer in terms of contaminants than inland sources.

- Avoid eating fish skin and trim visible fat, both of which may contain higher levels of contaminants.

- Younger, smaller fish are more likely to contain fewer contaminants than older, larger fish.

- Avoid eating the tomalley in lobster or the "mustard" in blue crab. This organ concentrates the contaminants within the seafood.

- Women of childbearing years should limit consumption of fatty fish. Bluefish, salmon, striped bass, swordfish, and freshwater fish, especially from the Great Lakes, can contain high levels of PCBs, which have been shown to be harmful to fetuses and infant development.

A toll-free national hotline has been established for individuals who want more information about seafood safety and preparation. Available weekdays from 9 A.M. to 5 P.M. Eastern Standard Time, the hotline number is 1-800-EAT-FISH.

All-American Eating

In standard restaurants and coffee shops, there are many options for nutritious meals. Consider oatmeal or poached or boiled eggs for breakfast. You can add a couple of slices of unbuttered whole grain toast. For lunch, soup and salad are still good mainstays. Hearty lentil, split pea, mushroom barley, black bean, and minestrone are satisfying and high in iron, B vitamins, and fiber. If necessary, you can skim the excess fat by dropping an ice cube into the soup, then skimming both the melting ice and fat that has been pulled to the surface. In hot weather, cold cucumber-yogurt or gazpacho soup fills the bill and provides valuable calcium. Main course salads such as Nicoise, Greek, or Waldorf (lemonize this one well because of the mayonnaise) are good luncheon fare, as are a chef's salad without the ham or a Cobb salad without the bacon and with less cheese.

Dinners can be built around any baked, broiled, grilled, or poached fish, seafood, chicken, beef, or lamb dish with steamed vegetables and salad. Healthful herbs like parsley and chives are often available for cooking or edible garnish. Since luncheons and dinners are nutritionally interchangeable, you can vary your meal's offerings, depending on your schedule.

Even fast-food restaurants offer some fairly nutritionally sound yet quick and convenient foods. A Taco Bell tostada is one of the lower fat items on a fast-food menu, with 30 percent of its calories from fat. Wendy's bowl of chili is even lower at 28 percent. A regular McDonald's hamburger *without* sauces and toppings is only 31 percent fat (add all the trimmings for a Big Mac and you have over 50 percent of the calories from fat!).

What about beverages with meals? Bottled mineral water or seltzer, including the newer fruit-flavored sparkling waters, is a cool, bubbling alternative to the calcium-leaching regular and diet soft drinks. Milk and milk-based drinks are important calcium sources. Fruit juices are widely available in most restaurants and can easily be diluted to 50 percent juice with the addition of water or sparkling water. Remember also that coffee or tea with a meal can inhibit iron absorption, and coffee increases calcium excretion. (If you cannot give up your coffee, at least save it for between meals when it is less harmful to your calcium and iron.) Steer clear of commercial iced tea mixes, although herbal teas are acceptable, unless candida is a problem, in which case avoid all teas. Many restaurants keep a selection on hand, or take your favorite herbal blends wherever you go. The Spicer's Bio Drink is also a good take-along and can be mixed with either hot or cold water (see Chapter Ten).

Ethnic Eating Advantages

Foreign cuisines provide many healthy and delicious eating options. Italian, Chinese, Mexican, French, and Japanese are America's current favorites, followed by Middle Eastern, Indian, and Thai. Trendy restaurants featuring Cajun and Creole cuisines are popping up all over the country.

Here's how you can get the most nutritional mileage from each one.

Italian

Make complex carbohydrates in the form of pasta or beans the highlight of your dinner. Pasta primavera (pasta with vegetables) or pasta with pesto (garlic, olive oil, parmesan, and pine nuts) or even linguine with red clam or mussel sauce are wonderful meal choices. Risotto (rice) and polenta (corn meal) may be featured in northern Italian cuisine.

A hearty bowl of minestrone or pasta/bean/vegetable soup can serve as a one-dish meal all by itself. Veal dishes, like veal marsala, piccata, or scallopini, are often deliciously prepared at Italian restaurants. Simply add a leafy green salad and sautéed vegetables. (Fresh vegetables usually abound in Italian cooking—sautéed peppers, zucchini, spinach, escarole, cauliflower, and eggplant.)

Escarole in chicken broth is my personal favorite as an appetizer. I also enjoy steamed or plain baked artichokes. No matter what I order, I always have several fresh lemon slices on the side to help emulsify any excess oil from whatever the source.

To avoid carbohydrate overload or gluten problems, skip the bread if you are having pasta.

Chinese

First, request that no monosodium glutamate (MSG), sugar, salt, or soy sauce be added during cooking. If you suspect an allergy to corn, also request that cornstarch be omitted. If peanut oil is used for cooking, choose light stir-fries of beef (flank steak is usually used), chicken, seafood, or tofu (bean curd), mixed with vegetables like bean sprouts, onions, water chestnuts, broccoli, scallions, bamboo shoots, and calcium-rich bok choy. Cellophane noodles made of rice or mung beans go well with small amounts of chicken, beef, tofu, or seafood in lo mein dishes (these are not choices for candida sufferers). Buddha's Delight, a vegetarian feast of mixed vegetables and noodles, is a favorite. I love eggplant in garlic sauce.

In general, Cantonese, which tends to have light sauces and crisp cooked vegetables, is a better choice than the heavier Szechuan or Hunan styles.

A word of caution. Watch for oyster and black bean sauces, which are highly salted. Ask for hot mustard, minced garlic, scallions, and some Chinese Five Spice from the kitchen instead.

Mexican

Tasty first courses include black bean soup, gazpacho, and guacamole seasoned with lots of fresh lemon and lime juice. Choose from entrees like chicken fajitas and chicken or shrimp with rice. Tortillas, which should be corn rather than flour because less lard is used, can be steamed rather than fried; even quesadillas can be griddle toasted instead of fried. Bean, chicken, or seafood burritos or enchiladas (minus the cheese), served with a dollop of sour cream and topped with lively salsa are good options. Vegetables like chilies, squash blossoms, jicama, and chayote cactus play a leading role in fine Mexican cuisine. Refried beans, however, are usually off limits because they are frequently made with lard.

French

France's cuisine boasts a wide variety of broiled, poached, and steamed foods. Selections such as fish en papillote, a traditional French favorite, is a delicious way to cook fish with herbs in its own juices. Other dishes such as bouillabaisse, coq au vin, poached salmon (without a heavy butter or cream sauce), and poulet aux fines herbes (roast chicken with herbs) are also suggested. Steamed mussels and that robust vegetable casserole, ratatouille, are also healthful menu selections.

Japanese

As with traditional Chinese fare, watch out for soy sauce. "Light" Japanese soy sauce is no less salty than regular soy sauce, just lighter in color. Also stay clear of teriyaki dishes (the sauce is a blend of soy sauce, saki, and sugar) as well as miso, a fermented soybean paste. Not only are these also high in salt, but all three items encourage yeast growth.

Japanese food has become synonymous with sushi. Raw fish is not recommended, no matter how meticulously prepared, because of the increasing levels of parasites and contamination being found in seafood at this time. However, sushi with avocado, cucumber, smoked salmon, or cooked crab or shrimp can be eaten safely. The green horseradish (wasabi) and pickled gingerroot accompaniments are strongly flavored condiments that are healthful additions. Noodle dishes with vegetables and chicken, steamed red snapper, grilled salmon or flounder are excellent selections. Calcium- and iron-rich hijiki seaweed is often braised in combination with mushrooms and carrots. Tofu-based soups made with kombu or wakame seaweed are safe bets (see Chapter Nine for more on versatile, healthful sea vegetables).

Other Ethnic and Regional Cuisines

In Middle Eastern and Greek restaurants, dips like hummus (garbanzo bean paté with sesame paste, garlic, and lemon) and babaghanoush (eggplant paté with sesame paste, garlic, and lemon) are served with pita bread. Used as an appetizer or salad dressing, these dips are good alone or cut with tzatziki (yogurt and cucumber). Side dishes of couscous (wheat-based pilafs) and rice-based pilafs can be found on the menu, along with tabbouleh, a grain salad of bulgur wheat, parsley, onion, tomatoes, mint, olive oil, and lemon. Greek salads or other feta cheese salads are wise nutrition choices. Shish kabob with meat and vegetables is also healthful.

If you go Indian, the pilafs and biryanis (rice-based

dishes) and dals (bean-based dishes) are delicious. The sweeter, nutty-flavored basmati rice may be on the menu. Chicken and lamb can be cooked Tandoori style in a clay oven, which seems to retain sufficient moisture, unlike broiling meat in a regular closed oven. Chicken or lamb korma with coriander and yogurt sauce makes a satisfying entree. If you like spicy-hot food, then vegetable and chicken curries will suit your taste. The dalia salad (bulgur, snow peas, and tomato with olive oil) is the Indian version of tabbouleh. Yogurt sauces and vegetables cooked in ghee (clarified butter) are permissible in small amounts. Pappadums (lentil wafers) are also permitted if they are baked, not fried. Chapatis and nan (garlic- or onion-accented bread) should also be baked, not fried. One item to watch is coconut, in the form of shredded garnish, oil, or milk used in cooking. These are high in saturated fat, the wrong kind of fat.

If you have discovered the unusual tastes of Cajun and Creole cooking, keep in mind "the simpler the better." Blackened redfish (minus the butter), shrimp or crab boil, chicken gumbo, shrimp creole, and seafood jambalaya (without the salt pork for sautéeing and ham and sausage for seasoning) fall within my guidelines.

In the Air

Most airlines are able to accommodate special diets if they are notified at least 24 hours ahead of schedule. Vegetarian, low sodium, or American Heart Association diet-based meals are usually available and, in many cases, are tastier than the standard fare, as well as healthier. Almost all the airlines offer a cold seafood plate that is relatively palatable. Delta Airlines offers breakfast muffins that are sweetened with fruit juice.

On the High Seas

Cruises are known for a number of things, one of which is the lavishness of their cuisine. If you are not careful, eating can become a full-time occupation on board, from early morning until late into the night. However, as with the airlines, you can request special diet menus if you notify the cruise line at least 24 hours before sailing. In addition, some cruise lines are preparing menu items more in line with the American Heart Association dietary guidelines.

As always, broiled, baked, or poached meats, poultry, and fish, accompanied by steamed vegetables and a fresh, green leafy salad, are healthful. Find an active partner and swim, walk around deck, attend lectures, or read, instead of succumbing to the desserts and snacks constantly available. A cruise, like any other vacation, can send you back to your daily existence refreshed and invigorated by the change of scene and pace; it need not send you back with candida, nutrient deficiencies, excess weight, dry skin and hair, and lowered immunity.

TWELVE

The Food-Wise Woman
Food Plan

We may live without poetry, music and art
We may live without conscience and live without heart
We may live without friends
We may live without books
But civilized man cannot live without cooks.

—Athenaeus, Greek writer

Supernutrition for Women has presented the most current information about the very special needs of a woman's body. Armed with your new knowledge, you have the best opportunity to make responsible choices about the food you will eat and how you will prepare it.

The key is to become an active "chooser," an active participant in life—rather than just a spectator. You can choose to create health or disease tomorrow by the living habits you practice today. Knowing that you can make a difference in your own health is the first step.

A Woman's Menu Planner and Recipe Guide

A well-prepared dish, according to an old Chinese saying, should appeal to the eye by its coloring, the nose by its aroma, the ears by its sound (crunch), and the mouth by its taste. We might add that for women who are concerned about health, a well-prepared dish should also contain high-quality protein, complex carbohydrates, essential fatty acids, and vitamins, as well as absorbable minerals such as calcium, iron, and other trace elements.

The following week-long menu plan and sample recipes show you how easy it can be to whip up nourishing meals. To highlight the variety possible on the plan, I've used different ingredients each day. However, you may want to repeat menus so that you are not left with too many leftover ingredients. Freeze muffins and breads so they are available and fresh when you want them.

I have included name brands when particular brands provide higher mineral levels or other nutritional benefits over other brands for a given product.

The daily calcium and iron totals are included at the end of each day's menu plan. These nutrients were computed with the assistance of Computrition, Inc. in Chatsworth, California, and *Agriculture Handbook* No. 8 from the U.S.D.A.

Items noted with an asterisk (*) appear in the recipe section that follows. You will also find several special recipes to introduce you to the flavor and versatility of mineral-packed sea vegetables.

Note: Choose from any of the following as beverages with your meals: herbal teas, mineral waters, or coffee substitute. Both regular tea and coffee inhibit calcium and iron absorption, so they should not be taken with meals.

Get ready, get set, enjoy.

Day One

Breakfast   1 small orange
1 egg scrambled with
1 ounce low-fat cheese (like Lifetime Swiss)
2 rice cakes with
2 tablespoons unsweetened apple butter
1 cup skim milk

Lunch   Black Beans with Olives and Cumin*
3 ounces canned salmon with
½ tablespoon canola mayonnaise
2 sesame bread sticks

Snack   2 ounces puffed millet
1 small pear with
½ cup non- or low-fat lemon yogurt

Dinner   Chopped parsley, tomato, and scallion with lemon juice dressing
4 ounces baked scrod with tarragon
½ cup steamed collards with
1 tablespoon sesame oil
1 small sweet potato

Snack   ¾ cup prune juice

Total calcium: 1,354 mg
Total iron: 16.5 mg

Day Two

Breakfast	½ cup low-sodium V-8 juice 1 baked corn tortilla with 1 ounce melted cheddar cheese (Lifetime brand) 1 cup hot carob drink made with skim milk
Lunch	1 cup nonfat milk 1 cup mushroom barley soup 1 oat bran muffin 1 small baked apple
Snack	½ cup non- or low-fat maple yogurt 4 halves dried apricots
Dinner	1 cup lentils with 1 teaspoon olive oil 1 cup steamed broccoli ¾ cup spaghetti squash with ½ cup marinara sauce and ¼ cup grated mozzarella cheese (Lifetime brand)
Snack	½ cup blueberries ½ cup non- or low-fat lemon yogurt

Total calcium: 1,784 mg
Total iron: 18.2 mg

Day Three

Breakfast   1 small banana with
½ cup non- or low-fat ricotta cheese
  (Calabro brand)
1 hard-cooked egg
½ cup skim milk

Lunch   1 cup steamed bok choy with red peppers
3 ounces baked garlic shrimp
1 cup brown rice with
1 tablespoon sesame oil and 2 tablespoons
  grated Parmesan cheese
Carrot and celery sticks

Snack   1 ounce Essence bread
1 tablespoon peanut butter

Dinner   4 ounces broiled lamb chop with rosemary
  and parsley
½ cup baked acorn squash with
1 teaspoon butter
1 cup steamed green peas

Snack   ½ cup non- or low-fat yogurt
½ cup apple-cranberry sauce

Total calcium: 1,170 mg
Total iron: 15 mg

Day Four

Breakfast
1 Fruity Fast Fizz* (with blueberries left
   from Day Two)
2 tablespoons blackstrap molasses
4 whole grain crackers

Lunch
3½ ounces salmon with salsa
½ cup grated raw beet, cabbage, and
   daikon salad with lemon juice dressing
1 cup cooked green beans
2 toasted rice cakes with
1 teaspoon butter

Snack
1 cup skim milk
2 ounces puffed kashi

Dinner
3 ounces lean ground beef burger, broiled,
   with sliced onions and parsley
Spinach salad with
1 ounce Lifetime cheese, crumbled, and
1 tablespoon safflower oil dressing
½ cup buckwheat groats
1 cup steamed zucchini and carrots

Snack
2 dates

Total calcium: 1,340 mg
Total iron: 13.8 mg

Day Five

Breakfast ½ small grapefruit
1 rice cake with
2 tablespoons almond butter and
1 tablespoon unsweetened raspberry preserves

Lunch 4 ounces canned tuna with celery, bean
sprouts, and water chestnuts mixed with
Handful blue corn chips
½ cup unsweetened pineapple chunks with
½ cup low-fat cottage cheese

Snack 1 cup non- or low-fat apple-cinnamon
yogurt with
2 ounces toasted wheat germ

Dinner ¾ cup macaroni and cheese
Cole slaw
1 cup cooked green split peas

Snack ½ cup unsweetened fruit cocktail

Total calcium: 1,983 mg
Total iron: 15.3 mg

Day Six

Breakfast 1 small nectarine
½ cup amaranth flakes
½ cup skim milk

Lunch Sassy Sardine Spread* on mini rice cakes
Celery, jicama, and cucumber rounds
1 cup cooked lima beans

Snack ½ cup non- or low-fat vanilla yogurt
2 dried apricot halves

Dinner 1 cup yogurt and pureed cucumber soup
with dill
Tossed salad with
1 tablespoon safflower oil dressing
3½ ounces shrimp with bean sprouts, bok
choy, and carrots

Snack 2 small plums

Total calcium: 1,263 mg
Total iron: 15.6 mg

Day Seven

Brunch   ½ cup cranberry juice cocktail
4 buckwheat pancakes with
8 tablespoons yogurt topping mixed with
1½ tablespoon blackstrap molasses
Hot carob drink made with skim milk

Snack   ½ cup ricotta cheese with
2 tablespoons toasted wheat germ

Dinner   Spiced Beef with Wine, Ginger, and
Garlic*
1 cup butternut squash
1 cup Mixed stir-sauteed greens with
1 tablespoon sesame oil dressing

Snack   1 cup non- or low-fat yogurt
4 tablespoons raisins

Total calcium: 2,311 mg
Total iron: 16.5 mg

Sample Recipes

Black Beans with Olives and Cumin

2 cups cooked black beans
2 scallions, finely chopped

4 large black olives, pitted and chopped
1 tablespoon virgin olive oil
4 tablespoons fresh lemon juice
1 teaspoon dried cumin
2 cloves garlic, mashed

Combine all ingredients in medium-sized bowl. Toss well. Can be served hot or cold as a side dish or as a salad on a bed of lettuce or mixed greens.
Serves 4   2.5 mg iron per serving

Fruity Fast Fizz

2 small ripe bananas
1¼ cup nonfat milk
¾ cup strawberries or ½ cup blueberries, blackberries, raspberries, or cherries

Place all ingredients in food processor or blender. Blend until smooth.
Serves 2   201 mg calcium per serving

Sassy Sardine Spread

1 4-ounce can sardines with bones, drained and flaked
½ cup nonfat or part-skim ricotta cheese (suggest Calabro brand)
½ cup green onions, finely chopped
1 teaspoon prepared white horseradish

Place sardines, cheese, green onions, and horseradish in bowl and mash together until well blended. Serve slightly chilled as an appetizer, light main dish, or snack with crackers or raw vegetables.

Serves 2 (6 tablespoons each)   400 mg calcium per serving

Spiced Beef with Wine, Ginger, and Garlic

1 pound flank steak, all visible fat removed
¾ cup dry red wine
4 teaspoons low-sodium Worcestershire sauce
    (available in health food stores)
1 teaspoon powdered ginger
4 cloves garlic, mashed

Place flank steak in baking dish and cover with mixture of wine, Worcestershire sauce, ginger, and garlic. Marinate for at least 2 hours in refrigerator.

Preheat broiler. Broil about 8–9 minutes on each side until done to preference. Serve hot from oven with salad and vegetable.

Serves 4   2.4 mg iron per serving

Tips to Boost Calcium in Your Diet

- Add 1 ounce crumbled feta cheese to the bottom of a bowl of soup. The cheezy flavor and billowing white swirls add pizzazz to any vegetable soup.

- Try 2 tablespoons prepared horseradish combined with ¼ cup nonfat cottage cheese and 2 tablespoons nonfat yogurt pureed in a blender for a quick sauce over steamed beets, rutabaga, or parsnips.

- When making soup stock, try to include the bones of chicken or beef to increase calcium content in the broth. One or two tablespoons of cider vinegar will help dissolve the calcium in these bones for better assimilation, without adding any vinegar taste.

- Choose dark leafy greens for your salads.

- A Caesar salad with extra cheese; a broccoli-cheese quiche; or a nog made with nonfat milk, egg yolk, crushed fruit and nuts will give you calcium and vitamins C and D in one dish.

- Choose sunflower seeds for a snack—one ounce has 3 times the calcium, 4 times the protein, and 9 times less sodium than one ounce of potato chips.

- Select herb teas that contain combinations of these calcium-rich herbs: parsley, kelp, burdock, borage, and chickweed, along with some of the more exotic ones like horsetail, Irish moss, capsicum, dulse, and comfrey.

- Use any of the following calcium-rich tidbits, alone or in combinations, to sprinkle over soups, salads, and casseroles or as snacks: toasted sesame seeds, sunflower seeds, soy granules, pistachio nuts or peanuts, parsley or red pepper flakes, kelp powder, horseradish, wheat bran or germ, dried lemon or orange peel. Sea vegetables like hijiki in soups and stew provide 14 times the calcium in a glass of milk.

- Remember that the nongluten grain quinoa has as much calcium as low-fat milk.

- While dairy products remain the best source for high calcium in a single serving, you don't have to take the high fat as well—buttermilk and low-fat or nonfat milk and yogurt are all high in calcium and low in saturated fats, as are goat's milk, acidophilus milk, and kefir for the lactose intolerant.

- Choosing part-skim milk mozzarella over cheddar saves you 45 calories per ounce and still gives you the calcium you want.

Tips to Get More Iron from Your Meals

- Since vitamin C enhances iron absorption, select appetizers prior to an iron-rich meal from items such as the following: tomato juice or soup, orange juice, citrus fruit salad cup, cantaloupe slice, or tomato and lettuce with basil-safflower oil dressing.

- Stuffed green peppers, made with lean ground beef, combine a vitamin C–rich food with an iron-rich one. Serve with tomato sauce and sprinkle with parsley and you add even more vitamin C.

- Cooking foods in large amounts of water can leach the iron from them, so steam vegetables to save their iron value.

- Pumpkin and sesame seeds are an iron-rich snack or garnish.

- The traditional cereal, milk, and fruit breakfast can be an iron booster by selecting strawberries, grapefruit, cantaloupe, or orange to accompany an iron-rich cereal. The milk will further increase iron absorption.

- Combine 1 tablespoon brewer's yeast with any of the following to make an iron-rich beverage: ½ cup tomato juice, ½ cup orange juice, or ½ cup skim milk with 1 tablespoon blackstrap molasses. Note that some people do experience diarrhea or intestinal pain when first trying brewer's yeast, so begin with ¼ teaspoon and work up to a tablespoon gradually. Also, since yeast overgrowth can be a problem, use these mixtures only as an occasional menu item.

- With as much iron as two eggs, a tablespoon of blackstrap molasses can be a valuable food source, despite its sugar drawbacks (see Chapter Five). Blend to a frothy mixture with a cup of skim milk or use it in place of jelly on an English muffin half.

- The preservative EDTA decreases iron absorption by as much as 50 percent from a given meal. Watch processed food labels and avoid this preservative when eating iron-rich foods.

Sea Vegetable Recipes

As I described in Chapter Nine, sea vegetables are a new and exciting way to get calcium, iron, and other nutrients women need. Agar agar, used instead of gelatin, has the added advantage of slowing down the absorption of sugar, avoiding the peaks and valleys of sugar consumption. Thus, it is a perfect addition to mousses and puddings. Hijiki, wakame, arame, agar agar, kombu, and nori are available in natural or health food stores. General instructions for preparation are included in Chapter Nine. These recipes were created for me by natural foods cooking expert, Eleonora Manzolini.

Molded Vegetable Gel

6 cups chicken or fish stock
5 tablespoons agar agar flakes
1 carrot, cut into ¼-inch slices
4 sprigs watercress
1 zucchini, cut into ¼-inch slices
½ cup arame, soaked in water for 15 minutes
½ cup corn kernels, boiled

Bring stock to a boil in soup pot. Sprinkle in agar agar flakes. Simmer until agar agar is dissolved, about 8–10 minutes. Arrange vegetables in a shallow 2-quart glass pan. Carefully pour liquid over vegetables. Chill until set.

Serves 4

Hijiki Noodles

1 pound whole wheat noodles, cooked and drained
¼ package hijiki seaweed, soaked in water and rinsed
    thoroughly
½ cup grated carrots
½ cup chopped celery
½ cup fresh minced parsley
½ cup minced scallions
1 clove garlic, minced
6 tablespoons extra virgin olive oil
    salt, pepper to taste

Combine vegetables and noodles. Toss with olive oil and seasonings. Let stand 30 minutes before serving.

Serves 6

Cucumber Wakame Salad

1 pound cucumbers, peeled and sliced
½ cup wakame seaweed, soaked in water for 15
    minutes, drained, rinsed, and coarsely chopped
1 tomato, cut into wedges
2 scallions, finely chopped
2 tablespoons sesame oil
1 tablespoon rice vinegar
1 teaspoon tamari

Combine cucumbers, wakame, tomatoes, and scallions. Mix the oil, vinegar, and tamari together. Toss the vegetable mixture with the oil mixture. Let stand 15 minutes before serving.

Serves 6

Carob Creme

4 cups unsweetened apple juice
5 tablespoons agar agar flakes
2 tablespoons carob powder
1 teaspoon vanilla extract
½ cup nonfat yogurt

Heat apple juice in a small saucepan over low heat. Sprinkle in agar agar and simmer until dissolved, about 8–10 minutes. Add carob and vanilla extract. Mix well with whisk. Pour into 1-quart shallow glass dish and chill until firm. Put set gelatin and yogurt in a blender or food processor and blend until creamy. Pour into individual serving dishes and refrigerate a few hours.

Serves 6

Lemon Mousse

6 cups unsweetened apple juice
1 teaspoon lemon zest
6 tablespoons agar agar flakes
    juice of 1 lemon
1 teaspoon vanilla extract
3 tablespoons tahini
6 lemon slices for garnish

In a saucepan, combine the apple juice, lemon zest, and agar agar. Bring to a boil and simmer until the agar agar is dissolved, about 8–10 minutes. Add lemon

juice and vanilla extract. Remove from heat and
let set. Blend with tahini until smooth. Pour into
individual serving cups. Garnish with lemon slices.

Serves 6

Strawberry Delight

3 cups nonfat milk
2¼ cups fresh strawberries, washed and hulled
¼ cup maple syrup
3 level tablespoons agar agar flakes
3 level teaspoons kuzu, diluted in 3 tablespoons cold
    water
¾ teaspoon vanilla extract
6 strawberries, sliced, for garnish
6 sprigs of fresh mint, for garnish

In a blender or food processor, blend milk and berries
until smooth. Combine in a saucepan with maple
syrup. Sprinkle in agar agar flakes and simmer 5–8
minutes, stirring occasionally. Add kuzu to pan while
stirring until thickened. Remove from heat. Add
vanilla extract. Divide into dessert cups and chill for 2
hours. Just before serving, garnish each with slices of
strawberries and a sprig of fresh mint.

Serves 6

More Ways to Free Food
from Fat, Salt, and Sugar at Home

For those of you who want to keep your current dietary
program, but need to make some minor changes in food
preparation techniques and choices to get the most nu-

tritional benefit from your diet, consider the following transitional ideas:

- Defat soups, stews, and stocks by chilling until the fat congeals and solidifies, then scrape off top layer before reheating.

- Broiling meats and poultry on a rack allows fat to drip off during cooking. Meatballs can be prepared this way, so that the excess fat drips into the pan under the rack, not into your sauce.

- If Tex-Mex or Southwestern cuisine is a family favorite, refried beans can be homemade without the lard and salt in commercial preparations. Simply rinse canned kidney beans and mash well with water, heat, and add hot spices like cayenne pepper, coriander, and cumin for flavor.

- Instead of frying tortillas for homemade enchiladas, dip them in tomato or enchilada sauce to soften them.

- For ethnic dishes usually requiring breading and frying, poach meat in wine, water, or broth, and then bake in a covered dish to retain moisture.

- To replace high-fat, high-salt sausage, use turkey or lean beef instead and add spices like garlic and fennel.

- Broccoli, zucchini, and spinach with Lifetime mozzarella make great pizza toppings instead of pepperoni or sausage. Veggies on pizza are one way to get children to eat their vegetables. Clients who have had to eliminate cheese from their diets because of lactose intolerance or genuine cholesterol problems tell me that they have discovered that pizza with tomato sauce, herbs, and lots of vegetables (but no cheese) can be as good or better than the traditional kind.

- To cut back on sodium, stock up on ready-made no-salt seasonings, such as No-Salt Mrs. Dash, Bell's Poultry Seasoning, Fines Herbs, Bouquet Garni, and Italian Herbs.

- Experiment with do-it-yourself herbs and spices, wines, and vinegars. Go ethnic with Chinese (mixture of ginger, coriander, and cayenne); northern Italian (wine vinegar and garlic); Indian (cumin, turmeric, curry, and coriander); Greek (lemon and oregano, or tomatoes and cinnamon); and French (wine, tarragon, and garlic).

- A fruit glaze can be tastefully used to frost cakes. Fruit-juice-sweetened apricot, peach, or strawberry preserves can be melted in a small saucepan, then spread warm on the cake.

- Freeze a low-fat fruit-flavored yogurt to make your own frozen yogurt.

- Try frozen bananas or grapes for a natural, cool dessert.

- Some people find chewing on a cinnamon stick helps them beat a sweet tooth.

- Instead of adding sweeteners to cereal grains, use aromatic crushed seeds like fennel, cardamom, anise, caraway, or coriander. One-half teaspoon ground anise or caraway seed adds a Scandinavian touch to cream of rye or rye berries cereal.

- Natural unsweetened applesauce is a good dessert choice. Mixed with 1 tablespoon raisins and a dash of cinnamon, it is a good snack or side dish.

- Lifestream Essene breads made from organically grown sprouts are delicious toasted in a pan in the oven. The natural sweetness from the sprouts will satisfy your sweet tooth. Plain or spread with natural apple butter, Lifestream breads make for a satisfying end of the meal.

Tips to Enhance Flavor

- Season after cooking for more flavor. Piping hot vegetables can be tossed or drizzled with herb mixtures and oil. Hazelnut oil adds a real gourmet touch to cooked green beans, brussels sprouts, broccoli, and snow peas.

- One half clove of well-minced garlic combined with 1 tablespoon of chopped parsley and onion goes a long way to perk up any hot vegetable combo—and may give added protection against yeast infections.

- Sauce up almost any dish with a lively salsa from south of the border. Combine 2 finely chopped medium tomatoes, ½ cup scallions, 2 tablespoons fresh or canned green chilies or jalapeño peppers, with 1 tablespoon red wine vinegar. Chill in the refrigerator before serving.

- Grilling vegetables provides a unique smokey flavor, which has made grilled vegetables so popular in the most trendy American restaurants. Just preheat your broiler for 15 minutes and glaze your favorite vegetables with olive, canola, or peanut oil. Cook for about 6 minutes, then turn them over and cook until tender.

- The flavor of millet is markedly increased when the grain is roasted similar to kasha or buckwheat groats. Just pan roast until the grain turns brown.

Making the Switch: Healthy Recipe Substitutions

My clients who are the most successful in achieving long-term benefits from my recommendations are those who incorporate small changes into their everyday eating patterns. There are many tasty ways to cut out excessive saturated and damaged fats, salt, sugar, refined carbohydrates, aluminum, and gluten from your recipes, so you can incorporate my recommendations without giving up flavor or your family's favorites. The chart below gives some tips for replacing recipe ingredients. To further reduce total fat and sugar intake, these substitutions reduce the fat by one fourth and cut the sugar by one half, which will not alter the taste of your prepared items.

In Place of:	Use:
1 cup margarine, shortening, or butter for baking	¾ cup canola or peanut oil
1 cup sour cream (47 fat grams)	1 cup low-fat yogurt (3.5 fat grams) or 1 cup buttermilk (2.2 fat grams) (To prevent yogurt separation when heating, mix 1 tablespoon yogurt with 1 tablespoon of cornstarch, stir into 1 cup yogurt, and heat until thickened.)
1 tablespoon cream cheese (5.3 fat grams)	1 tablespoon kefir cheese (3 fat grams)
2 tablespoons butter mixed with 1 tablespoon flour for sauce and soup thickener (7 fat grams)	2 tablespoons arrowroot, potato starch, or kuzu (0 fat grams)

In Place of:	Use:
1 cup whole milk yogurt (7.4 fat grams)	1 cup low-fat yogurt (3.5 fat grams) or nonfat yogurt (0.4 fat grams)
1 cup whole milk (8.2 fat grams)	1 cup 1 percent (low-fat) milk (3.5 fat grams) or nonfat milk (0.4 fat grams)
cream in sauces	equal quantities of evaporated skim milk (Keep heat low; it curdles if boiled.)
cream in soups	⅓ cup pureed beets, potatoes, and carrots to 2 cups simmering soup
Parmesan or Romano cheese	lemon zest and garlic
1 tablespoon sugar for cooking	½ tablespoon honey, molasses, or pure maple syrup
1 cup sugar for baking	½ cup honey (If you are using as much as ¾ cup honey, then decrease other liquid by ¼ cup for each ¾ cup honey. If there is no liquid in recipe, then add ¼ cup flour for each ¾ cup honey. Also, lower the baking temperature by 25 degrees; honey and molasses tend to caramelize at higher temperatures.)
1 tablespoon cocoa	1 tablespoon carob powder
1 ounce or square baking chocolate	3 tablespoons carob powder + 1 tablespoon water + 1 tablespoon oil

In Place of:	Use:
1 cup wheat flour for baking	1 cup corn flour; ¾ cup coarse cornmeal; ¾ cup + 3 tablespoons fine cornmeal; ½ cup + 2 tablespoons potato starch flour; ¾ cup + 2 tablespoons rice flour; 1 cup soybean flour + ¼ cup potato starch; 1 cup millet meal (Non-wheat flours need 10 to 20 minutes more baking time.)
1 tablespoon wheat flour	½ tablespoon cornstarch; ½ tablespoon potato starch; ½ tablespoon rice flour; ½ tablespoon arrowroot; 2 tablespoons quick-cooking tapioca; 1 tablespoon millet meal
1 cup white rice	1 cup brown rice (Increase cooking time by 20 minutes if cooked alone, 30 minutes if combined with other foods.)
1 teaspoon salt during cooking	½ teaspoon kelp powder after cooking
baking powder, regular (containing aluminum)	equal quantity of aluminum-free baking powder (Royal, Rumford, Price, Schillings), low-sodium and cereal-free by Cellu or Featherweight

In closing, may I wish that all of you who have read this book and are applying its principles enjoy a lifetime of quality longevity. As my grandfather Aaron used to say, "May you live till 120!"

Selected References

Books

Appleton, Nancy. *Lick the Sugar Habit*. Garden City Park, NY: Avery Publishing Group, 1988.

Atkins, Robert C., and Shirley Linde. *Dr. Atkins' Super-Energy Diet*. New York: Crown Publishers, 1977.

Burkitt, Denis. *Eat Right to Stay Healthy*. New York: Arco, 1979.

Coffey, Lynette. *Wheatless Cooking*. Berkeley, CA: Ten Speed Press, 1986.

Connolly, Pat, and Associates of the Price-Pottenger Nutrition Foundation. *The Candida Albicans Yeast-Free Cookbook*. New Canaan, CT: Keats Publishing, 1985.

Cooper, Kenneth H. *Controlling Cholesterol*. New York: Bantam Books, 1988.

———. *Preventing Osteoporosis*. New York: Bantam Books, 1989.

Crook, William G. *The Yeast Connection*, 3rd edition. Jackson, TN: Professional Books, 1986.

Dalton, Katharina. *Once a Month*, 3rd rev. ed. Claremont, CA: Hunter House, 1987.

Eck, Paul C. and Wilson, Larry. *Toxic Metals in Human Health and Disease*. Phoenix, AZ: The Eck Institute of Applied Nutrition and Bioenergetics, Ltd., 1989.

Edelstein, Barbara. *The Woman Doctor's Medical Guide for Women*. New York: Morrow, 1982.

Erasmus, Udo. *Fats and Oils: The Complete Guide to Fats and Oils in Health and Nutrition*. Bonita, CA: Gerson Institute, 1986.

Fardon, David F. *Osteoporosis, Your Head Start on the Prevention and Treatment of Brittle Bones*. New York: Macmillan, 1985.

Frederick, Carlton. *Carlton Frederick's Guide to Women's Nutrition*. New York: Putnam, 1988.

Gittleman, Ann Louise. *Beyond Pritikin*. New York: Bantam Books, 1988.

Hausman, Patricia. *The Calcium Bible*. New York: Rawson Associates, 1985.

Hills, Hilda Cherry. *Good Food, Gluten Free*. New Canaan, CT: Keats Publishing, 1985.

Horrobin, David F. *Clinical Uses of Essential Fatty Acids*. Montreal: Eden Press, 1982.

Hunt, Douglas. *No More Cravings*. New York: Warner Books, 1987.

Hunter, Beatrice Trum. *Gluten Intolerance*. New Canaan, CT: Keats Publishing, 1987.

——. *The Sugar Trap and How to Avoid It*. Boston: Houghton Mifflin, 1982.

Kunin, Richard A. *Mega-Nutrition for Women*. New York: McGraw-Hill, 1983.

Lansky, Vicki. *The Taming of the C.A.N.D.Y Monster*. New York: Bantam Books, 1982.

Lesser, Michael. *Nutrition and Vitamin Therapy*. New York: Grove Press, 1980.

Long, Patricia. *The Nutritional Ages of Women*. New York: Macmillan, 1986.

Lorenzani, Shirley S. *Candida: A Twentieth Century Disease*. New Canaan, CT: Keats Publishing, 1986.

Marks, Betty. *The High-Calcium, Low-Calorie Cookbook*. Chicago: Contemporary Books, 1987.

Niazi, S. K. *The Omega Connection*. Oakbrook, IL: Esquire Books, 1987.

Ojeda, Linda. *Exclusively Female. A Nutrition Guide for Better Menstrual Health*, 2nd edition. Claremont, CA: Hunter House, 1983.

Page, Melvin E., and H. Leon Abrams, Jr. *Your Body Is Your Best Doctor*. New Canaan, CT: Keats Publishing, 1972.

Pfeiffer, Carl. *Mental and Elemental Nutrients*. New Canaan, CT: Keats Publishing, 1975.

Pinckney, Edward, and Cathey Pinckney. *The Cholesterol Controversy*. Los Angeles: Sherbourne Press, 1973.

Polivy, Janet, and P. Herman. *Breaking the Diet Habit: The Natural Weight Alternative*. New York: Basic Books, 1985.

Rawcliffe, Peter, and Ruth Rolph. *The Gluten-Free Diet Book*. Englewood Cliffs, NJ: Prentice-Hall, 1985.

Reading, Chris M., and Ross S. Meillon. *Your Family Tree Connection*. New Canaan, CT: Keats Publishing, 1988.

Reuben, Carolyn, and Joan Priestley. *Essential Supplements for Women*. New York: Perigee Books, 1989.

Rosenvold, Lloyd. *The Gluten Connection*. Hope, ID: Rosenvold Publications, 1988 (available from P.O. Box 330, Hope, ID 83836).

Seid, Roberta Pollack. *Never Too Thin*. Englewood Cliffs, NJ: Prentice-Hall, 1989.

Truss, C. Orian. *The Missing Diagnosis*. Birmingham, AL: C. Orian Truss, M.D., 1982 (available from P.O. Box 226508 Birmingham, AL 35226).

U.S. Department of Agriculture. *Composition of Foods, Fats and Oils, Raw, Processed, Prepared*. USDA Agricultural Handbook No. 8-4, 1979.

———. *Nationwide Food Consumption Survey. Continuing Survey of Food Intake by Individuals*. NFCS, CSFII Report No. 86-1, 1986.

Wallach, Leah. *Food Values: Calcium*. New York: Harper & Row, 1989.

Whitlock, Evelyn P. *The Calcium Plus Workbook*. New Canaan, CT: Keats Publishing, 1988.

Yudkin, John. *Sweet and Dangerous*. New York: P. H. Wyden, 1972.

Periodicals

Abraham, Guy E. and Ruth E. Rumley. "The Role of Nutrition in the Management of the Premenstrual Tension Syndromes." *Journal of Reproductive Medicine*, vol. 32, number 6, p. 405, June, 1987.

Adler, Andrew J., Ruth Shainkin-Kestenbaum, and Geoffrey

M. Berlyne. "Aluminum Absorption and Intestinal Vitamin D Dependent Ca Binding Protein." Abstract, *Kidney International*, vol. 37, p. 471, 1990.

Anderson, James W., Linda Story, Beverly Sieling, Wen-Ju Lin Chen, Marilyn S. Petro, and Jon Story. "Hypocholesterolemic Effects of Oat Bran or Bean Intake for Hypercholesterolemic Men." *American Journal of Clinical Nutrition*, vol. 40, p. 1146, 1984.

Bjorksten, J., L. Yaeger, T. Wallace, and coworkers. "Control of Aluminum Ingestion and Its Relation to Longevity." *International Journal for Vitamin A and Nutrition Research*, vol. 48, p. 462, 1988.

Bland, Jeffrey, Ph.D. "Break the Cycle of Monthly Discomfort." *Delicious*, March 1988.

———. "Building Stronger Bones." *Delicious*, July/August 1988.

———. "Candid Talk About Candida." *Delicious*, November/December 1988.

Brown, Michael H. "Here's the Beef: Fast Foods Are Hazardous to Your Health." *Science Digest*, April 1986.

Brownell, Kelly. "The Yo-Yo Trap." *American Health*, March 1988.

Bullen, Beverly A., Gary S. Skrinar, Inese Z. Beitins, Gretchen von Mering, Barry A. Turnbull, and Janet W. McArthur. "Induction of Menstrual Disorders by Strenuous Exercise in Untrained Women." *New England Journal of Medicine*, vol. 312, p. 1349, 1985.

"Can Aluminum Cause Alzheimer's?" University of California, Berkeley Wellness Letter, October 1986.

Carr, C. J., and Ralph Shangraw. "Nutritional and Pharmaceutical Aspects of Calcium Supplementation." *American Pharmacy*, February 1987.

Cooper, Kenneth H. "The Calcium Controversy." *Family Circle*, February 21, 1989.

Cowley, Geoffrey. "Cholesterol Confusion." *Newsweek*, September 18, 1989.

Curatolo, Peter W., and David Robertson. "Health Consequences of Caffeine." *Annals of Internal Medicine*, vol. 98, p. 641, 1983.

Dyerberg, J., H. O. Bang, E. Stoffersen, S. Moncada, and J.

R. Vane. "Eicosapentaenoic Acid and Prevention of Thrombosis and Atherosclerosis?" *Lancet*, vol. 2, p. 117, 1978.

Eaton, S. Boyd, and Melvin Konner. "Paleolithic Nutrition." *New England Journal of Medicine*, vol. 312, p. 283, 1985.

Forgang, Isabel. "Heart Association Nutrition Expert Says Entire Generation May Be at Risk." *San Diego Union*, June 28, 1987.

Fox, Arnold. "Your Calcium Bank." *Let's Live*, May 1984.

Gaby, Alan R. "Cholesterol Confusion." *Pathways/DC Resources*, Spring 1985.

"The Golden Age of Natural Oils." *Delicious*, April 1988.

Grundy, Scott M. "Comparison of Monosaturated Fatty Acids and Carbohydrates for Lowering Plasma Cholesterol." *New England Journal of Medicine*, vol. 314, p. 745, 1986.

Heaney, Robert, and Robert R. Recker. "Effects of Nitrogen Balance, Phosphorus, and Caffeine on Calcium Balance in Women." *Journal of Laboratory and Clinical Medicine*, vol. 99, p. 46, 1982.

Hepburn, Frank N., Jacob Exler, and John L. Weihrauch. "Provisional Tables on the Content of Omega-3 Fatty Acids and Other Fat Components of Selected Foods." *Journal of the American Dietetic Association*, vol. 86, p. 788, 1986.

Ince, Susan. "Indulgence and Denial." *Self*, March 1989.

Jibrin, Janice, and Randall Fuller. "The United Tastes of America." *Self*, March 1989.

Kaplan, Janice. "Exercising Bones." *Vogue*, March 1989.

Liebman, Bonnie. "Is Dieting a Losing Game?" *Nutrition Action Healthletter*, March 1987.

———. "The All-American Junk Food Diet." *Nutrition Action Healthletter*, May 1988.

McGrath, Mike. "Can Calcium Lower Blood Pressure?" *Prevention*, April 1988.

Mihalik, Maria. "Who Gets Anemia?" *Prevention*, November 1986.

Neilson, F. H., Hunt, C. D., Mullen L. M., Hunt Jr. "Effect of Dietary Boron on Mineral, Estrogen and Testosterone Metabolism in Postmenopausal Women," *Applied Science of Experimental Biology*, vol. 1, pg 394–397, 1987.

Nicar, Michael J., and Charles Y. C. Pak. "Calcium Bioavailability from Calcium Carbonate and Calcium Citrate." *Journal of Clinical Endocrinology and Metabolism*, vol. 61, p. 391, 1985.

Popkin, B.M., Haines, P.S., and Reidy, K.C. "Food Consumption Trends of U.S. Women: Patterns and Determinants Between 1977 and 1985." *American Journal of Clinical Nutrition*, vol. 49, p. 1307, 1989.

Prasad, Anada S., Donald Oberleas, K. Y. Kei, Kamran S. Moghissi, and Joanne C. Stryker. "Effects of Oral Contraceptive Agents on Nutrients: I. Minerals." *American Journal of Clinical Nutrition*, vol. 28, p. 377, 1975.

Quint, Laurie, and Bonnie Liebman. "Putting Calcium into Perspective." *Nutrition Action Healthletter*, June 1987.

Recker, Robert R. "Calcium Absorption and Achlorhydria." *New England Journal of Medicine*, vol. 313, p. 70, 1985.

Roblin, Andrew. "Clean Out Your Cholesterol." *Prevention*, October 1988.

———. "Splash on the Olive Oil and Cut Your Cholesterol." *Prevention*, January 1989.

Sorlie, Paul, Tavia Gordon, and William B. Kannel. "Body Build and Mortality: The Framingham Study." *Journal of the American Medical Association*, vol. 243, p. 1828, 1980.

Späetling, L., and G. Späetling. "Magnesium Supplementation in Pregnancy: A Double-Blind Study." *British Journal of Obstetrics and Gynecology*, vol. 95, p. 120, 1988.

Squires, Sally. "Being Alert to the Good Fish and the Bad." *Washington Post Health*, April 4, 1989.

"The Stanford University Guide to a Healthier Heart." *Prevention*, February 1986.

Taylor, C. B., S. K. Peng, N. T. Werthessen, P. Tham, K. T. Lee. "Spontaneously Occurring Angiotoxic Derivatives of Cholesterol." *American Journal of Clinical Nutrition*, vol. 32, p. 40, 1979.

Weinstock, Cheryl Platzman. "The 'Grazing' of America: A Guide to Healthy Snacking." *FDA Consumer*, March 1989.

Witkin, Steven S. "Defective Immune Responses in Patients with Recurrent Candidiasis." *Infections in Medicine*, May/June 1985.

Appendix A

Guide to Reducing Dietary Fat

This guide shows the amount of fat in diets with different proportions of calories from fat. For example, a 2,000 calorie diet calculated to have 30 percent of calories from fat has a total of 67 grams of fat, or 600 calories from fat. Food labels can help you find how many grams of fat are contained in packaged foods.

Percent of Calories Desired From Fat	Total Calories From Fat Should Not Exceed	Total Grams of Fat Should Not Exceed
For a 1,500 calorie diet:		
40 percent	600 calories	67 grams
35 percent	525 calories	58 grams
30 percent	450 calories	50 grams
25 percent	375 calories	42 grams
20 percent	300 calories	33 grams
For a 2,000 calorie diet:		
40 percent	800 calories	89 grams
35 percent	700 calories	78 grams
30 percent	600 calories	67 grams
25 percent	500 calories	56 grams
20 percent	400 calories	44 grams

Percent of Calories Desired From Fat	Total Calories From Fat Should Not Exceed	Total Grams of Fat Should Not Exceed
For a 2,500 calorie diet:		
40 percent	1,000 calories	111 grams
35 percent	875 calories	97 grams
30 percent	750 calories	83 grams
25 percent	625 calories	69 grams
20 percent	500 calories	55 grams

Source: Public Health Service, National Institutes of Health, *Diet, Nutrition and Cancer Prevention: A Guide to Food Choices* (NIH Publication No. 85-2711, November, 1984).

Appendix B

Fat and Calories from Some Foods

If you choose to reduce the fat in your diet to 30 percent of your daily calories, for a 2,000 calorie diet that is about 67 grams of fat.

Food	Serving	Calories	Grams of Fat
Dairy Products			
Cheese:			
American, pasteurized process	1 oz	105	9
Cheddar	1 oz	115	9
Lifetime Cheddar	1 oz	65	3
Cottage:			
Creamed	½ cup	115	5
Low-fat (2%)	½ cup	100	2
Cream	1 oz	100	10
Mozzarella, part skim	1 oz	80	5
Lifetime Mozzarella	1 oz	60	2
Parmesan	1 tbsp	25	2
Swiss	1 oz	105	8
Lifetime Swiss	1 oz	60	3
Cream:			
Half and half	2 tbsp	40	3
Light, coffee, or table	2 tbsp	60	6
Sour	2 tbsp	50	5
Ice Cream	1 cup	270	14

Food	Serving	Calories	Grams of Fat
Ice Milk	1 cup	185	6
Milk:			
Whole	1 cup	150	8
Low-fat (2%)	1 cup	125	5

Dairy Products

Food	Serving	Calories	Grams of Fat
Nonfat, skim	1 cup	85	trace
Yogurt, low-fat, fruit-flavored	8 oz	230	2

Meats

Food	Serving	Calories	Grams of Fat
Beef, cooked:			
Braised or pot-roasted:			
Less lean cuts, such as chuck blade, lean only	3 oz	255	16
Leaner cuts, such as bottom round, lean only	3 oz	190	8
Ground beef, broiled:			
Lean	3 oz	230	15
Regular	3 oz	245	17
Roast, oven cooked:			
Less lean cuts, such as rib, lean only	3 oz	225	15
Leaner cuts, such as eye of round, lean only	3 oz	155	6
Steak, sirloin, broiled:			
Lean and fat	3 oz	250	17
Lean only	3 oz	185	8
Lamb, cooked:			
Chops, loin, broiled:			
Lean and fat	3 oz	250	17
Lean only	3 oz	185	8
Leg, roasted, lean only	3 oz	160	7

Food	Serving	Calories	Grams of Fat
Pork, cured, cooked:			
Bacon, fried	3 slices	110	9
Ham, roasted:			
Lean and fat	3 oz	205	14
Lean only	3 oz	135	5
Pork, fresh, cooked:			
Chop, center loin:			
Broiled:			
Lean and fat	3 oz	270	19
Lean only	3 oz	195	9
Pan-fried:			
Lean and fat	3 oz	320	26
Lean only	3 oz	225	14
Rib, roasted, lean only	3 oz	210	12
Shoulder, braised, lean only	3 oz	210	10
Spareribs, braised lean and fat	3 oz	340	26
Veal cutlet, braised or broiled	3 oz	185	9
Sausages:			
Bologna	2 oz	180	16
Frankfurters	2 oz (1 frank)	185	17
Pork, link or patty, cooked	2 oz (4 links)	210	18
Salami, cooked type	2 oz	145	11

Poultry Products

Chicken:			
Fried, flour-coated:			
Dark meat with skin	3 oz	240	14
Light meat with skin	3 oz	210	10

Food	Serving	Calories	Grams of Fat
Chicken, roasted:			
Dark meat without skin	3 oz	175	8
Light meat without skin	3 oz	145	4
Duck, roasted, meat without skin	3 oz	170	10
Turkey, roasted:			
Dark meat without skin	3 oz	160	6
Light meat without skin	3 oz	135	3
Egg, hard cooked	1 large	80	6

Seafood

Food	Serving	Calories	Grams of Fat
Flounder, baked:			
With butter or margarine	3 oz	120	6
Without butter or margarine	3 oz	85	1
Oysters, raw	3 oz	55	2
Shrimp, french fried	3 oz	200	10
Shrimp, boiled or steamed	3 oz	100	1
Tuna, packed in oil, drained	3 oz	165	7
Tuna, packed in water, drained	3 oz	135	1

Grain Products*

Food	Serving	Calories	Grams of Fat
Bread, white	1 slice	65	1
Biscuit, 2½ inches across	one	135	5
Muffin, plain, 2½ inches across	one	120	4
Pancake, 4 inches across	one	60	2

Food	Serving	Calories	Grams of Fat
Other Foods			
Avocado	½	160	15
Butter, margarine	1 tbsp	100	12
Cake, white layer, chocolate frosting	1 piece	265	11
Cookies, chocolate chip	4	185	11
Donut, yeast type, glazed	one	235	13
Mayonnaise	1 tbsp	100	11
Oils	1 tbsp	120	14
Peanut butter	1 tbsp	95	8
Peanuts	½ cup	420	35
Salad dressing:			
Regular	1 tbsp	65	6
Low calorie	1 tbsp	20	1

Source: Human Nutrition Information Service, U.S. Department of Agriculture. For fat and calorie values for other foods, see *Nutritive Value of Foods*, HG-72, for sale from Superintendent of Documents, U.S. Government Printing Office, Washington, DC 20402.

*Most breads and cereals, dry beans and peas, and other vegetables and fruits (except avocados) contain only a trace of fat. However, spreads, fat, cream sauces, toppings, and dressings often added to these foods do contain fat.

Notes

Chapter 4

1. Gaby, Alan, M.D., "Cholesterol Confusion," *Pathways*, (Washington, D.C.: D.C. Resources, 1989) p. 58.
2. C. B. Taylor, et al. "Spontaneously Occurring Angiotoxic Derivatives of Cholesterol." *American Journal of Clinical Nutrition*, 1979, 32:40–42.
3. S. E. Langer, *Solved: The Riddle of Illness* (New Canaan, CT: Keats Publishing, 1984) p. 99.
4. "Cholesterol-Proofing Food," *American Health*, March 1989, p. 22.
5. Robert C. Atkins and Shirley Linde, *Dr. Atkins' Super-Energy Diet* (NY: Crown, 1977) p. 230.
6. *Prevention*, November 1986, p. 106.

Chapter 6

1. Jane Brody, *Jane Brody's Nutrition Book* (NY: Bantam Books, 1987) p. 95.
2. Shirley S. Lorenzani, Ph.D., *Candida: A Twentieth Century Disease* (New Canaan, CT: Keats Publishing, 1986) p. 26.
3. Cited in: William G. Crook, M.D., *The Yeast Connection* (Jackson, TN: Professional Books, 1986) p. 315.
4. Lorenzani, p. 74.
5. G. S. Moore and R. D. Atkins, *Mycologia*, 1977, 69:341.
6. Cited in: Crook, p. 275.

Chapter 7

1. Cited in: Beatrice Trum Hunter, *Gluten Intolerance* (New Canaan, CT: Keats Publishing, 1987) p. 12.
2. Hilda Cherry Hills, *Good Food, Gluten Free* (New Canaan, CT: Keats Publishing, 1986).

Chapter 8

1. H. Spencer, et al., *Gastroenterology*, 1975, 68:990.
2. Evelyn Whitlock, M.D., *The Calcium Plus Workbook* (New Canaan, CT: Keats Publishing, 1988) p. 7.
3. Jeffrey Bland, "Building Stronger Bones," *Delicious*, July/August 1988, p. 12.
4. Ibid.
5. Whitlock, p. 15.
6. *American Pharmacy*, February 1987, NS27 (2):49.
7. *The New England Journal of Medicine*, 1985, 313:70.

Chapter 9

1. Michael Lesser, M.D., *Nutrition and Vitamin Therapy* (NY: Grove Press, 1980) p. 108.
2. Richard Kunin, M.D., *Mega-Nutrition for Women* (NY: McGraw-Hill, 1983) p. 5.
3. L. Späetling and G. Späetling, "Magnesium Supplemen-

tation in Pregnancy: A Double-Blind Study," *British Journal of Obstetrics and Gynecology*, 1988, 95:120.
4. Guy E. Abraham and Ruth E. Rumley, "The Role of Nutrition in the Management of the Premenstrual Tension Syndromes," *Journal of Reproductive Medicine*, June 1987, 32:6:405.

Chapter 11

1. Quoted in "Being Alert to the Good Fish and Bad," *Washington Post Health*, April 4, 1989, p. 9.

Index

Abraham, Guy, 140
Acidophilus (Lactobacillus acidophilus), 91, 173
Additives in food, 149, 205
Adelphi University, 55
Adrenal gland, 82, 137
  hormones, 82
Aerobics Center, Dallas, 49
Agar agar. *See also* Recipe Index, 144
Agriculture Handbooks, 126n
Ahrens, Edward, 52
Airline food, 190
Allicin, 91
Alpha-linoleic acid. *See* Omega 3
Aluminum, 23, 27, 113, 114–115

antacids with, 114–115, 117
  cooking and, 114, 178–179
  health hazards, 178
  label reading and, 154
  sources, 114, 154
    beverage cans/containers, 154
    in food, 154
    nonfood items, 154
    soft drinks, 154
Alzheimer's disease, 27, 178
Amaranth, 103, 104
American
  calcium deficiencies, 110
  candy consumption, 62–63
  cholesterol levels, 33
  cuisine, 184–186

Recipe Index

ABOUT THE AUTHOR

Ann Louise Gittleman, M.S., has an extraordinary background in both traditional nutrition and holistic health. After graduating from Connecticut College, and studying at the New York Institute of Dietetics, she obtained a master's degree in nutrition education from Columbia University.

Since then, she has maintained a private practice for over thirteen years with clients nationwide. Ann Louise served as the Chief Dietitian of the Pediatric Clinic at Bellevue Hospital in New York City, Bilingual Nutritionist for the USDA's Women, Infants, and Children Food Program at a Yale University-connected Health Clinic in New Haven, Connecticut, and as Nutritional Consultant for the first holistic medical group in Connecticut, Deep Brook Associates, which was headed by Dr. John Rhinehart.

Prior to writing her first book, *Beyond Pritikin,* Ann Louise was Nutrition Director at the Pritikin Longevity Center in Santa Monica, California. After leaving the Pritikin Center, she has been a consultant to various nutritionally oriented medical doctors, corporations, and environmental health clinics. She is the chairman of the Department of Nutrition of the American Academy of Nutrition, a member of the American Nutritionists Association, the Holistic Meidcal Foundation, and the World Research Foundation. She has been a frequent guest on nationwide television and radio and has been interviewed by national newspapers and magazines.

J. Lynne Dodson is a full-time freelance writer with over twenty years' experience in medical and health care communications. She has been on the editorial staff of several medical journals, including *World Journal of Surgery* and the *Journal of Electrocardiology*, and helped prepare numerous books for publication such as *Medicine and Its Technology* and *The Origins of the American Corporation*. Her educational materials on nutrition and health have been used in schools throughout the nation.

Ms. Dodson is currently writing a resource book and newsletter for new physicians on how to establish and operate a private practice.